Walk Away
the
Pounds

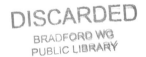

Walk Away
the
Pounds

The Breakthrough Six-Week Program
That Helps You Burn Fat, Tone Muscle,
and Feel Great Without Dieting

Leslie Sansone
with Rowan Jacobsen

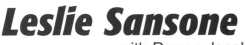

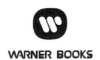

WARNER BOOKS

NEW YORK   BOSTON

Neither this exercise program nor any other exercise program should be followed without first consulting a health-care professional. If you have any special conditions requiring attention, you should consult with your health-care professional regularly regarding possible modification of the program contained in this book.

Warner Books

Time Warner Book Group
1271 Avenue of the Americas, New York, NY 10020
Visit our Web site at *www.twbookmark.com*.

Walk Away the Pounds is a registered trademark of GT Merchandising & Licensing LLC.

Printed in the United States of America

First Printing: January 2005
10   9   8   7   6   5   4   3   2   1

Library of Congress Cataloging-in-Publication Data

Sansone, Leslie.
Walk away the pounds : the breakthrough 6-week program that helps you burn fat, tone muscle, and feel great without dieting / Leslie Sansone with Rowan Jacobsen.
p. cm.
ISBN 0-446-57700-6
1. Fitness walking. 2. Weight loss. 3. Reducing exercises. I. Jacobsen, Rowan. II. Title.
RA781.65.S23 2005
613.7'176--dc22
                                                2004008740

Book designed by Mada Design, Inc.

WALKING IS MAN'S BEST MEDICINE.

— HIPPOCRATES

CONTENTS

PART I

THE HEART
OF THE MATTER

SHE WALKS IN BEAUTY, LIKE THE NIGHT
OF CLOUDLESS CLIMES AND STARRY SKIES;
AND ALL THAT'S BEST OF DARK AND BRIGHT
MEET IN HER ASPECT AND HER EYES . . .

— LORD BYRON

1. Walk Away Those Pounds!

Congratulations! By picking up this book, you have already made a statement about what you value in life. You've taken one small step away from being a couch potato or a desk potato, and one step toward a life of looking great, feeling great, and taking charge of your goals. True, it's only one small step, but that is how you start. In this book I'll teach you how to take more and more steps.

Most of the things I'll show you are so simple that you won't even realize you're taking steps until you look back and see how far you've come. Sound too good to be true? Quite the opposite. As I've been showing people for twenty-five years, it's as easy as putting one foot in front of the other.

Walking is a miraculous thing. We tend to take it for granted, but just look at a toddler. When she takes those first wobbly steps, that look on her face is pure magic. It says, Gee, this is fun! It says, I'm one of you now! And it says, This is exactly what I should be doing! We human beings are designed to walk—and walk a lot. So many factors in our modern lifestyle—cars, remote controls, desk jobs—work against that, but you'll be amazed by how many good things fall into place once you make walking a regular part of your life. Fat melts away. Clothes fit. Food tastes better. Health problems disappear. Mood improves. Sex is more fun. Energy levels soar. Sleep becomes deep and satisfying. Stress evaporates. As it is for a toddler, life becomes something to embrace each morning, rather than a daily grind. And this is all because of exercise.

If exercise can do all this for us, then why doesn't everybody get some? Well, that is the bone I have to pick with the modern fitness industry. Watching those ultrafit pros do their intense workouts has never been terribly inspiring to me. I know that kind of body requires hours of dedication every day—and who has that kind of free time? Walking is my business, but you know what? I *still* need to squeeze my exercise in around driving the kids to baseball and softball practice, finding the pet lizard that has escaped his cage again, putting a nutritious dinner on the table, and being at my best for the meetings, public events, and decisions that make up my work life.

And here's the secret. It isn't hard to fit exercise in, because you don't need hours a day. You don't need six-pack abs. You aren't auditioning to be a stunt double in the next *Charlie's Angels.* Just give yourself fifteen minutes a day, for starters, and all the benefits will follow: the trimmer tummy, tighter muscles, lower blood pressure, reduced stress levels, and the satisfied feeling at the end of the day, knowing that you took another step forward.

I can't tell you how many hundreds of women have written to me, telling me the stories of how they lost real weight—twenty pounds, forty, sixty, even one hundred—following my walking program. You'll meet many of them in this book, hear their stories, and see their transformations. Starting by walking just one mile— or less—these women walked away the pounds and kept them off. I think the reason so many women have success with my system is because it is so easy, so gentle, yet so effective. You don't have to be coordinated. You don't have to learn any complicated poses or routines. You just put one foot in front of the other and walk, walk, walk.

THE PERFECT EXERCISE

When I began teaching aerobics classes in the 1980s, I didn't set out to change the way people exercise. I just taught the dance-aerobics programs I had learned. But over time, I gravitated toward walking and developed my own program, because that was what worked for almost everyone, regardless of size or fitness level. No matter how out of shape they were when they started, people lost weight through walking and became healthier and happier in the process.

What is it about walking that makes it more successful than other exercises? Part of it is the simplicity. Everyone can walk. It's so easy, in fact, that some people are skeptical about whether you can really get in shape by just walking. But studies are confirming what I've suspected all along: walking is *excellent* exercise. According to the *New England Journal of Medicine*, walking just thirty minutes a day, three times a week, reduces the risk of death from all natural causes by 55 percent! Walking also keeps you in the midrange of aerobic activity, where fat oxidation is most efficient. That's right: You burn more fat through low-intensity sports like walking than through intense activities that leave you gasping for breath, such as weight lifting or high-energy aerobics. Not only that but you also continue to burn fat *after* walking. And once you've been walking for a few weeks, you'll have raised your metabolic rate, so that you burn more calories all the time, even when you're sitting or sleeping!

Then there are the things that don't happen when you're walking. You don't crash. You don't get injured. You don't compete against someone else.

You also don't go broke. Too many people are hesitant to start exercising because they think it will be expensive and intimidating. Many people don't want to invest in fancy home equipment and aren't comfortable in a fitness club environment. Not a problem. Just lace up a decent pair of sneakers in your living room and you are ready to walk.

I didn't begin teaching with the concept of in-home walking, either. Again, that developed from teaching thousands of women and discovering what worked for them and what held them back. Having to drive to a fitness club to exercise keeps many people from doing it regularly. So does trying to do exercises that are too difficult. So does bad weather. Walking outside can be wonderful, but suddenly it rains for a week, you skip your walks, your energy sags, and the next week you find excuses not to get back to it. There is always a day when it's too hot outside, too

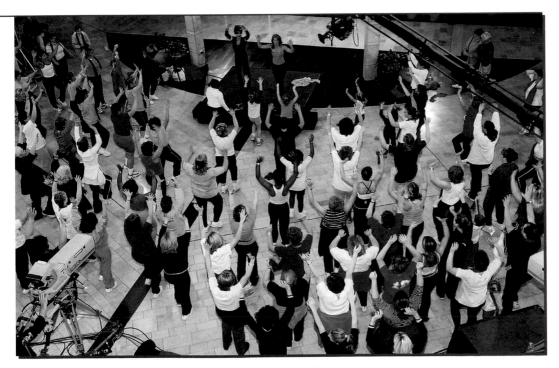

My pal Jackie Zeman loves to get out there and lead walks with me!

cold, or when you don't want to deal with the dogs, the bugs, the traffic lights, or the car fumes.

But your living room is always the right temperature for walking. And when you don't have to worry about making forward progress, you can use my specially formulated series of moves—side steps, knee lifts, and so on—to work a much wider range of muscles than you can by walking around the block. Whether you use my videos for company, your favorite music, or a buddy, you'll find that the half hour you set aside for walking is a part of the day you always look forward to.

THE PAYOFF

What You'll Typically Achieve After Six Easy Weeks

Fat: ↓ 15 pounds
Muscle: ↑ 5 pounds
Looks: Fab!
Metabolism: ↑ 200 calories every day—not including your exercise!
Risk of heart disease: ↓ 45 percent
Risk of stroke: ↓ 42 percent
Blood pressure: ↓ 10 points
Total cholesterol: ↓ 10 percent
Good (HDL) cholesterol: ↑ 5 percent
Risk of diabetes: ↓ 58 percent
Overall risk of early death: ↓ 55 percent
Husband: Watches Y-O-U instead of E-S-P-N*
Children: Loving, obedient, and supportive*

*Some models may vary.

DO IT FOR LOVE

Before you hop up and start walking off those pounds, let's talk about motivation. You bought this book, which means you're ready to change your life. But are you really interested in a healthy lifestyle, or are you trying to fit into those old pants for your high school reunion in two months? If you're doing it for the pants, that's okay! Many people begin a diet or exercise program with an immediate goal of changing their looks, often for a specific event. If that's what it takes to get you started, great. But most everyone who loses weight for looks puts it back on again later. The reunion ends, the swimsuit season is over, and you slip back to your old habits. Worse still, if you lost weight through some sort of crash diet, your metabolism slows down, you burn fewer calories, and you gain the weight back even though you stuck to the diet.

On the other hand, people who lose weight for better health, rather than looks, tend to keep it off. Unlike a reunion, health is an ongoing part of our lives. And people who lose weight for health do it because they care about themselves. They know that overweight people die sooner and are more susceptible to disease, and they want to make sure they lead full, rewarding lives. This kind of self-love can be one of the strongest supports in your life.

And don't forget your children, your spouse, your friends and relations. Keeping healthy, so that you stick around longer, have more energy, and face life with a sunnier outlook, is one of the best ways to show your love to those most important to you.

Do it because you love life, too. Your life is a gift from God, and all you have to do to return the favor is simply be a good steward of that life. (Boy, you should see my kids scatter when Mom starts one of her preachfests!) Whatever your beliefs are, you have been given an amazing gift—the chance to live a life on this planet. It would be a shame to waste it sitting on the couch.

My Story

I remember perfectly when the revelation hit me that simply moving one's body could be a way of celebrating life, of tapping in to the essence of what it means to be alive and part of creation. I certainly didn't grow up knowing that. I didn't exercise any more than most girls did in the seventies.

Back when I was eighteen and took my first aerobics class, if you had told me that my career would be in aerobics, I would have laughed all the way to my architectural-engineering course. I was a freshman in college, you see, and that was my major. But I came from a working-class Pennsylvania family; there was no money to send the kids to college, so if I was going to make it, I had to support myself.

The work ethic in my family was strong. While growing up, I'd always worked. I was the girl who asked you if you wanted fries with your burger at McDonald's. I cleaned houses and baby-sat. So I looked around for a job in Pittsburgh, where I was going to school, and answered an ad for something called California Aerobic Dance. Instructors were needed—no experience necessary. I didn't even know what aerobics was. But I took a weekend seminar, and it was like somebody had stuck smelling salts under my nose. *It felt so good to be moving!* After the class, I felt energized, healthy, and I was in a good mood for hours. I wanted more! I eagerly became an instructor. Along the way, I lost the extra "freshman fifteen" I was carrying. Weight loss had never been my goal, but I immediately noticed how good I felt once the excess pounds came off!

In 1979, I taught my first aerobics class. It was California Aerobic Dance, just as I'd learned it. Seeing it excite other people, too, and seeing them change before my eyes was the best feeling in the world. My enthusiasm must have been infectious, because people kept coming back for more. I felt that it was my duty to spread the good word about fitness to as many people as I possibly could, so I would go to rec centers, church halls, you name it—anywhere I could set up my boom box and Maxwell

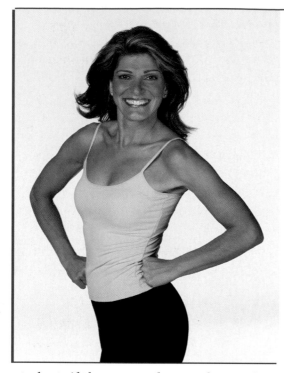

House coffee can. (I didn't want anyone to be kept away because they couldn't afford to come, so I just put out a can for donations.)

I made enough money to keep myself in college—and then some. I'll never forget the day I came home from a half-hour class at my own church, dumped $150 out of the coffee can onto my bed, and watched my mother's face turn ashen. "What did you do to earn this money?" she cried. When I told her it was from teaching aerobics, she was even more astonished than I was.

Before long, all my classes were filled. I couldn't possibly teach additional classes and still have time for college, so I started asking my best students if they wanted to teach, too. Soon I had fifteen instructors working for me, fanned out across the church halls of Pittsburgh and New Castle. The logistics were nuts! After a few years, we had turned into a real business—but with no office!

In 1985, I opened Studio Fitness and got all the classes under one roof. The type of aerobics we taught was still dance-based, but I became more and more aware of a problem. Not everyone was comfortable with the fast-paced dance steps we used. We were thriving, but we were losing some people—often the very people I knew could benefit the most from my program. Something had to change.

One late-October day, I was driving around, pondering this dilemma. It was a classic Pennsylvania fall day, cold and blustery, with dry leaves skittering across the sidewalks. I happened to notice a group of walkers bustling past me. Good for them, I thought, even on this chilly day. But what would they do in a month or two, when the snows came? Hard to keep up an exercise program if you had to shelve it four months of the year.

Bingo! That very day, I drove back to the studio and placed a tiny ad in the paper for an introductory WalkAerobics class. I knew that brisk walking could raise people's heart rates enough to deliver the same benefits as dance aerobics. I knew it wouldn't be everybody's cup of tea, I just hoped we would get the fifteen or twenty students needed to cover costs. Well, when I walked into that studio room a few days later, there were ninety people waiting to take the class! I had tapped into a vein I didn't even know existed.

Over the next year, we filled *forty* WalkAerobics classes a week. Woman after woman came up to tell us how she hadn't thought she could ever do an aerobics class until she saw our ad. These same women were now doing many miles each week. Every day, I went home feeling gratified by what we were doing.

One day, a student who had to miss a class asked if she could tape the class. So we taped it, and suddenly everyone wanted copies of the tape so they could do extra sessions at home. The second lightbulb went on.

We contacted every video distributor, and one responded enthusiastically right away. The man who owned it was also Italian, and he teased me. "What's this little Italian girl doing walking?" he asked. As a matter of fact, Italians are big walkers. Go to Florence or Rome right now and see what everyone is doing in the evening. They're eating their gelato and walking the streets and plazas of the city, people watching. There's no better entertainment on a summer's evening. Unfortunately, European cities are a lot more walker-friendly than American cities, so we have to be creative about getting our walks in.

The distributor picked us up, and the rest is history. With no advertising whatsoever, we took off. Why? Remember that this was the era of Jane Fonda's workout tapes: the perfect bodies, the skintight leotards, the acrobatic moves. A lot of people couldn't relate.

But here we were. Whatever we were about, it seemed real! We had bodies of all shapes and sizes up there on those videos, walking. Our choreography was sketchy, and our leg warmers didn't even match, but we were walking and having a darned good time doing it. That was something everyone could relate to. And somehow we managed to be more popular than Jane in certain quarters.

Twenty years later, we're still at it, still giving people new tools (like this book!) to help them achieve their goals. I am so thankful that I've had the chance to meet so many of my students and to spread the word to millions of women that staying active and feeling great is not just for jocks and models; it's for all of us, large and small, rich and poor, mother, daughter, and grandmother, too.

THEIR STORIES

What makes my work so fulfilling to me, day in and day out, are the women I hear from, those whose lives I have touched in some positive way. There is no better feeling in this world than having someone come up to you and say that they have turned their lives around, and that you had some small role to play in that. On the following pages are the stories of two women who had the courage to take charge of their health.

Walking Wonder

Jill Cooley
RALEIGH, NORTH CAROLINA

Lost 140 pounds

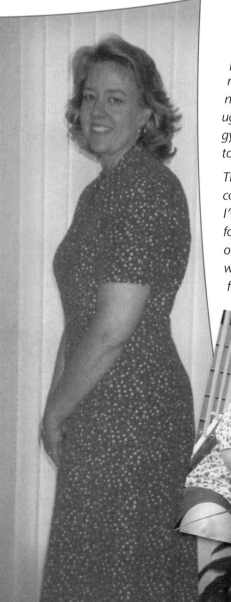

In August 2001, I began my weight-loss journey. I weighed 290 pounds, felt miserable, and hated what I saw in the mirror. Approaching 300 pounds and taking blood pressure medication, I knew it was time for a change—not just another diet but a whole lifestyle change. With a mountain of determination and lots of prayer for strength, I began making healthier food choices and moderating my portions. But I knew changing my diet alone would not get me where I wanted to be. Yes, the dreaded word reared its ugly head: exercise! At my weight, I felt too embarrassed to go to a gym, and all the exercise videos that were suggested to me seemed too complicated or intimidating.

Then I saw a commercial for Walk Away the Pounds. Well, I knew I could do something as simple as walking, so I thought I'd give it a try. I've been walking with Leslie ever since! The basic steps were easy to follow, Leslie was energetic and upbeat, and her walkers were women of all shapes and sizes. Gradually, I worked my way up from one-mile walks to three-mile ones with hand weights. And the pounds began to fall off. Family, friends, and coworkers were (and still are) amazed! In March 2003, I reached my goal of 155 pounds. I have maintained my program and even lost additional weight. My family is very proud of me, and, yes, I am proud of myself. I've even got my mom walking with Leslie now! At thirty-nine years old and five eight, I look better, feel better, and like myself better than I can ever remember.

Walking Wonder

Julie Probus-Schad

Wentzville, Missouri

It wasn't until I was admitted to the hospital to rule out a cardiac event that I realized I had to take control of my health if I wanted to be around to participate in life with my loved ones. In the hospital, I was given a stress test on a treadmill. I was never so embarrassed in my life! At age thirty-six, I could barely last a few seconds, let alone the time needed to get an accurate reading. Fortunately, I had not had a cardiac event, but I did have another serious health problem: obesity. My sedentary lifestyle had allowed me to balloon up to 218 pounds.

Lost 80 pounds

I started my weight-loss journey with Weight Watchers and by walking outside, but after a few walks in the dead of winter, I heeded my Weight Watchers leader's advice and purchased Walk Away the Pounds. At first, walking for five minutes winded me. But the positive attitude expressed in the program is very uplifting. Seeing people of all fitness levels with the common goal of improving their health is truly an inspiration. Soon, I was not only losing pounds but, more importantly, losing inches and increasing my stamina. The cardiovascular benefits were amazing! My health improved immensely.

Today, I have lost eighty pounds and thirteen inches off my hips. My cholesterol was 256 and is now in the normal range. I enjoy the walking; it is not a burden. Knowing I can do one mile or four is encouraging because I set the pace, depending on my schedule. I am able to keep up with my ten-year-old and have so much more energy. I am truly a new woman.

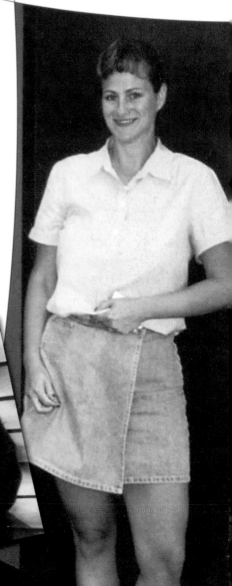

Julie and Jill turned their lives around by simply making the decision to take that first step. You'll meet many more Walking Wonders like them in this book. If you identify at all with these women, if you've ever found yourself in one of those ruts where you had lost sight of your goals, where you didn't like what was happening to your body and spirit but were so far down in that rut that you couldn't see your way out of it, then you are one of the people I hope to reach with this book. The way out is simpler than you ever could have guessed. You simply walk right out of that rut. But on your journey to healthy living, you need to know where to go, so think of this book as your map. Follow it to some places that can really help you on your journey. Those places include learning about aerobic exercise and strength training, healthy lifestyle habits, and how to avoid some of the traps that the modern world sets for us. But the most important place we'll visit on this journey is not a place we usually associate with fitness. It's the house of the spirit—*your* spirit. Caring for your spirit, letting it thrive and grow as you reach your goals and set new ones, gives you a foundation for all your strength in life. And it just so happens that the body is the temple for that spirit. You wouldn't let your community church fall to ruins. It's just as important to keep your own temple in the glorious condition in which it was made. Do that and it will always be filled with a divine and vital spirit that emanates out to every part of your life and the lives of all those you touch.

2. The Whats and the Whys

❖ **WHAT DO I GET IN** *WALK AWAY THE POUNDS*?

A unique six-week program that combines in-home walking, simple strength training, motivational breakthroughs, and commonsense advice to help you burn calories, lose fat, firm muscles, reduce stress, avoid illness, shake off the blues, and boost your energy levels sky-high. Beginners get a simpler approach to fitness, one that will change their lives.

Those already doing my videos will find a complete system to integrate their workouts into the rest of their lives, using their new energy and self-esteem to find fulfillment.

❖ **WHY WALKING?**

You may not be able to master underwater sumo wrestling, advanced yoga for invertebrates, or whatever the latest fitness craze is, but that "one foot in front of the other" thing is a no-brainer. And studies show that walking is the perfect exercise to get your heart in that midlevel aerobic range, where you burn fat most efficiently.

❖ **WHAT IS AEROBIC EXERCISE?**

Exercise that lasts more than a few minutes and gets your heart rate up, using the oxygen you breathe to burn fat calories for energy. Walking, running, biking, swimming, and tennis are all aerobic. Weight lifting and sprinting aren't. Aerobic exercise is the best thing you can do for your heart, your lungs, and your waistline.

❖ WHAT ARE THE HEALTH BENEFITS?

Following this program will *dramatically* reduce your risk of heart disease, high blood pressure, stroke, depression, osteoporosis, and diabetes. It will also have a significant impact on your risk of arthritis, cancer, back pain, asthma, emphysema, and Alzheimer's disease. Are you walking yet?

❖ WHY IN-HOME WALKING?

Walking in place allows you to use a wide range of steps, so you work all your muscles, not just a few. You can exercise right in the comfort of your living room, at any time of day you want. Job schedule, kid schedule, and weather are never a problem. Your chatty neighbor won't stop you for twenty minutes. You can reach your fitness goals while watching TV. Is this exercise paradise, or what?

❖ WHAT IS STRENGTH TRAINING?

Strength training involves *anaerobic* exercises that build muscle, such as weight training and Pilates. Any exercise that involves working against resistance—either gravity or extra weight—counts. Strength training doesn't provide much cardiovascular benefit, but it's even better at toning muscle and improving bone strength than aerobic exercise is. When combined, they form two sides of a golden coin. You do the strength training part of my program while you walk, so it takes no extra time at all.

❖ WHAT EQUIPMENT WILL I HAVE TO BUY?

Nothing—provided you already own a pair of sneakers. To do my program, you need no fancy machines, weights, or outfits of any kind. Some people like to use inexpensive pedometers to track their steps; others time themselves. You can buy some hand weights or a stretch band to do upper-body exercises, or can use something you have at home, such as filled water bottles. You can walk in your underwear. Hey, you can even walk in your birthday suit! Don't tell me—just lower the blinds and walk!

❖ WHAT KIND OF AWFUL DIET ARE YOU GOING TO MAKE ME EAT?

People rarely lose weight permanently with food diets alone; they yo-yo instead. And they don't get the amazing health benefits that come from exercising. Yes, healthy eating is a vital part of long-term health and weight control, but it isn't as important as the exercise component, and too many people do nothing because they have had bad diet experiences. That's why I recommend an exercise "diet."

❖ What if I am already on a diet?

My program is flexible enough to work with whatever diet program you follow. In fact, if you are already dieting and then you add my walking program to your routine, you'll be *stunned* at how much faster the weight disappears. This is why so many people using Weight Watchers and other diet plans begin walking with me. I actually recommend doing it the other way around, though: Start walking *before* you tinker with your diet. Once you've made exercise a habitual part of your life, your body will automatically desire better food, and eating healthy—or sticking to your favorite diet—will come naturally.

❖ Why six weeks?

Experts know that if you can do something for twenty-one days, you internalize it as a new habit. At that point, it becomes more of a mental effort to break the habit than to keep doing it. After six weeks, not only do you have a healthy habit for life but you have been exercising long enough to see real differences in weight, muscle tone, cholesterol level, blood pressure, and mood.

❖ What if I already do your videos?

One of the main reasons I created this book was because I heard from so many walkers who used my videos but wanted more structure and guidance. They wanted a *program* that would help them continually improve. They also found that their walking success made them pay attention to other aspects of their lives, such as stress and nutrition. "Give us a road map, Leslie," they said, and that's what I've tried to do here. The basic program in this book is designed for beginning walkers. For those who prefer using videos, I provide recommendations each week of the program for videos that match the walking and strength-training routines for that week. If you already use my videos several days a week, you should use my chapter "PowerWalking: The Advanced Program for Current Walkers" to design walks appropriate for you. Be sure to combine these walks with my Walk Boosters, motivation strategies, nutrition tips, and stress guide to get the maximum health and emotional benefits.

❖ What if I don't have any videos?

You don't need them. The walking moves are very simple; I demonstrate them all in the book. To track distance indoors, you can either time yourself with a clock or use a pedometer to count steps. You can design your own program around outdoor walks, your favorite TV show, or music.

❖ WHAT IF I GET BORED?

Remember that TV thing? You can use one of my videos and walk with me, or you can tune in the Discovery Channel and walk with the penguins. Either way, it beats walking around the same old block.

TEN MYTHS ABOUT EXERCISE

1. I'm too out of shape to exercise.

This myth keeps way too many people on the couch. Listen to me, friend: It is never too late to exercise! The trick is to start slowly, which is what my program does. You may be amazed to discover how easily it comes!

2. To get real health benefits, I have to exercise strenuously.

Actually, moderate exercise, such as walking, delivers the best health results. Exercising to the point of exhaustion burns less fat, suppresses the immune system, and discourages people from continuing. In a recent study at the University of Miami, people who walked thirty minutes per day lost just as much weight as people who walked sixty minutes.

3. I don't have the time to exercise.

Think about how you spend your days. Do you read the paper in the morning? Do you sleep in? Do you plunk down after work and unwind with a glass of wine? Do you watch TV every evening? We all make choices about how to spend our time. Considering you can devote as little as fifteen minutes a day to my program and still get results, you are *choosing* whether you want health and happiness or not. Besides, the extra energy you get from walking lets you get more done in your day, not less.

4. Exercise will make me eat more.

If you're gaining weight, you already eat more than your body needs. Daily walking regulates your appetite. You learn to eat only what you really need. That's why I say that when you start on the Walk Diet, everything else takes care of itself!

5. Exercise is expensive.

Getting sick is expensive. Visiting doctors and taking drugs for diabetes, high blood pressure, and high cholesterol is expensive. Staying healthy through walking is cheap, cheap, cheap.

Whatever you want it to be. If getting fit makes you fall in love with the world all over again, and reminds you of the special place you hold in creation, then hallelujah! If my program just makes you break out the bathing suit and strut down the beach, then hallelujah for that, too.

---

6. Exercise will leave me feeling exhausted.

Just the opposite. Gentle exercise will leave you energized and enthusiastic. Again: You'll accomplish more, not less.

7. I'm older, so why bother exercising now?

Older adults are the people who can benefit the most from exercise! All the health problems associated with aging—brittle bones, weight gain, muscle loss, poor balance, even mental decline—can be arrested or even *reversed* with regular exercise.

8. Exercise is dangerous for my heart.

Not exercising is dangerous for your heart. Unless you already have serious heart concerns or push yourself to the point where you collapse in a puddle on the ground, your heart is at no additional risk from walking. It will be one of the first organs to thank you for keeping it active.

9. My problem is depression. Exercise can't help me with that.

Your mind and body are intimately connected. Study after study have shown regular exercise to be just as effective as drugs in lifting mild to moderate depression—with no side effects (unless you count weight loss). And it doesn't take weeks to kick in, either. If you feel down, *make* yourself exercise immediately and see if it does the trick.

10. I don't like that bulky look people get from working out.

That's why walking is such a beautiful thing. You get all the health, mood, and weight-loss benefits of other exercises, but instead of looking like the Terminator, you look your slim, trim, feminine best!

3. The Miracle of Exercise

Hi there. Come right into Dr. Leslie's office and have a seat. What's troubling you? Weight control? I've got just the prescription for you. It's rigorously tested, absolutely safe, and incredibly effective.

What's that? You've got high blood pressure, too? Well, this prescription also happens to work for that. It will even improve your cholesterol at the same time.

How about you? Diabetes? This same prescription should help control that, too. And you, come right in and lie down on Dr. Leslie's couch. Feeling depressed? I'm going to prescribe the same medicine for you.

Insomnia? It should help with that, too. And once you're over the depression, I recommend a maintenance dose from now on, because it helps prevent cancer, arthritis, osteoporosis, heart disease, and stroke.

There are some side effects, of course. You'll probably feel more energetic and less stressed. There will be some weight loss. Your memory could improve. And you'll start to look really good. But you'll have to live with that.

The cost? No charge. This is one prescription you can fill for free.

The miracle drug I'm talking about isn't new, of course. And it isn't a medicine at all—at least not in the traditional sense. It's exercise. But if it could be prescribed as a pill, in the words of Robert Butler, M.D., founder of the National Institute on Aging, "it would be the single most widely prescribed drug in the world." No other substance or activity can improve your mental and physical life in so many ways.

Yet half the adults in the United States

choose not to take it, leading to hundreds of thousands of preventable deaths each year. If a new blood pressure medication were responsible for this, it would be front-page news and special task forces would be created to remedy the situation.

Actually, presidents have created task forces to get people to exercise, but even these haven't helped much. Our culture of video games and drive-through windows doesn't help, either. One of the strangest things about the modern world is that we have come to think of exercise as something separate from regular life. Sure, a few of us carry boxes or paddle kayaks for a living, but most of us hardly burn an extra calorie during our workdays. We drive, we sit, and we take an elevator up to the office. And in the evenings, we don't even get up to change channels anymore! This change is more recent than you might realize.

Not so long ago, most kids still walked to school. People lived in small enough communities that adults could walk to work, to market, or wherever they had to go. Most folks still worked on farms, where exercise was part of the job from dawn to dusk. Even in big cities, people would walk twenty blocks without thinking about it, and they often walked up four or five flights of stairs to their apartments.

In just a few generations, this has all changed. Elevators, cars, taxis, and takeout have all become more prevalent in our lives. The most hyped invention of the past twenty years was Segway, a machine designed solely to keep people from having to walk!

The problem is, the human body is an even more glorious design, and it was *made* for walking. For proof, look at those two masterpieces of engineering sticking out from your hips and connecting you to the ground. They have only one purpose. If we were designed for a life of sitting, we'd look like one of those blow-up clowns that you can't knock over—no legs, all middle, with maybe a cup holder built into one's belly button.

And that is practically what we become if we don't exercise. "Use it or lose it" is more than a slogan. Your body does a wonderful job of molding itself to meet your needs. It simply gives you what it thinks you want. If you spend no time exercising but every evening sitting on your backside watching *CSI*, your body thinks, Hmmm, guess I don't need to make any more muscle if it won't be used, but some extra padding down there might be really comfy! If, on the other hand, you walk every day, your body feels those muscles contracting, that miraculous heart pumping, and thinks, Hey! This would be even easier with more muscle. More oxygen! More blood! And it gives you what you need.

If you have good silver, you know better than to keep it stored away and use it only once a year. It just gets tarnished sitting in the drawer. But regular use keeps it at its beautiful, gleaming best. Your most precious possession of all—your body— works the same way.

This is why I say exercise is the best medicine we have. It literally causes the body to make more good stuff—more muscle, more enzymes, more bone, more blood. At the same time, exercise causes you to store less fat because you use the energy from your food to move instead. You become toned and trim. Best of all, exercise triggers a cascade of chemical changes in the body, all designed to keep you functioning as an active human being should. If you are going to be an active person in the world, you need energy and stamina, can't get sick much, need to live a long time, and need to feel happy as you look forward to each day. By exercising and eating right, you give your body the raw material it needs to deliver on all these requirements. You signal to it the type of life you plan on leading, and it gives you what you need to live that life. It's a beautiful, wonderful feedback loop. And the only way it doesn't work is if you don't try.

WHAT YOU GET FROM EXERCISE

I know, facts can be boring—and I promise to keep things short—but if you're like me, you'll enjoy learning about the amazing changes in store for you as you walk off the pounds, the blues, the sleepies, and health concerns of all kinds. And if you have a husband who's skeptical that walking is great exercise, or a friend you're trying to convince to walk with you, just hand 'em these pages. They'll be up alongside you in no time.

Weight Loss

Let's face it: The number-one reason people start exercising is to look better. You know it works; the differences between active and inactive people are obvious—not just toned muscles and lack of fat, but skin tone and healthy glow, too. You don't need me to tell you about it. What I do want to tell you is that exercise is essential to *any* weight-loss plan. A survey of women who had lost weight and kept it off found that 86 percent had used exercise to do so. As I discuss later, dieting alone rarely works in the long run; even all the leading food diets—such as South Beach, Atkins, and Weight Watchers—recommend an exercise component like my program.

While I hope that weight loss is just step one in your plan for a more active and fulfilling life, if looking good is your only goal, that's fine, too. Vanity is an excellent motivator. There are vain reasons to exercise, and healthy reasons to exercise. The beauty of it is that it doesn't matter which you choose—you get all the benefits either way! I don't care *why* you exercise, as long as you do it. Exercise to look great, and feel lucky later on when you find yourself staying healthy into old age. Or exercise for your health, and be pleased when friends start exclaiming over how great you look.

Everyone knows they can lose weight by exercising more; what they want to know is how much to exercise. Obviously, this depends on how much weight you need to lose to begin with. The more overweight you are, the more quickly you can shed pounds by getting back on your feet. I've heard from plenty of women who lost 100 pounds or more by doing my videos and eating right, but that won't happen (and shouldn't!) if you weigh 160 to begin with. I work with women of all shapes and sizes, but the average woman I hear from weighed 150 to 160 pounds when she began my program and achieved her goal of losing 10 to 15 pounds. Consider that a *very* realistic goal.

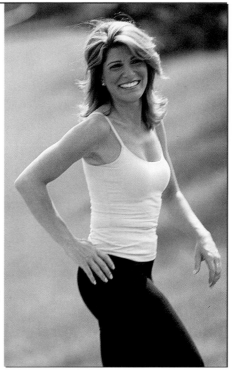

Heavenly Bodies

We've all had friends who looked dramatically different after following a fitness routine for as little as a few weeks. "Gosh," we say to them, "you look like you've lost a ton of weight!" They probably have lost a little weight, but what we are really noticing is how much tighter their bodies look and how much better they carry themselves.

The toning comes from burning up fat by exercising and replacing it with new muscle. Muscle weighs more than fat, and, as we all know, fat hangs all over the place, while muscle keeps its shape, so a body with 10 percent more muscle and 10 percent less fat will actually weigh more but will look thinner, stronger, and better.

Posture also makes a huge difference. Most of us slouch. But regular walking makes us more attractive from day one by requiring us to stand up and tuck our tails in. That gives us an extra inch or two, gets everything back in its proper place, and allows us to move and lift without discomfort. And that is the goal, because it's not about some number on a scale; it's about how your new body looks and about all the things you can do with it that you couldn't do with the old model.

Cholesterol and Blood Pressure

When I talk to the women who follow my fitness program, I ask what it was that finally made them say, "Enough is enough! I've got to get fit." I hear all kinds of answers. Sometimes it was just a certain glance in a mirror, or a certain comment from a husband. Sometimes it was a friend who inspired them. Maybe it was a half-mile walk that became an ordeal. Often they come to exercise under doctor's orders. "Lose weight or you're going to develop diabetes." "Lose weight or I'm putting you on hypertension medicine." And most common of all: "If you can't lower your cholesterol through a diet and exercise program, I'm going to have to put you on medication."

Conditions such as high cholesterol and high blood pressure are major factors in developing cardiovascular disease, the number-one killer in America, accounting for 39 percent of natural deaths. Fortunately, they are also the conditions most improved by aerobic exercise. One recent study found that women who walk just one hour per week reduce their risk of heart attack. That's right: Just get up, do one mile with me four times per week, and you've already improved your long-term health. Keep walking through my six-week program, and you'll have cut your chance of developing heart disease by an incredible 45 percent! Your chance of having a stroke will also go down by 42 percent. Of course, you have to keep walking if you want to maintain the benefits.

Several exercise factors are responsible for protecting your heart. When you exercise, your blood vessels dilate to allow more blood to flow through them and deliver oxygen to your muscles. This regular dilation—and the accompanying contraction of the vessels after exercise—helps keep them flexible and clean, which keeps your blood pressure down and prevents cholesterol from sticking to them. When cholesterol sticks, it starts to create blockages that prevent the blood from flowing. A blockage on the way to the heart results in a heart attack. A blockage on the way to the brain results in a stroke. The blood vessels also get bigger through regular workouts, meaning there is less flow and pressure in them the rest of the time. Overall, half the people taking blood pressure medication were able to stop after beginning moderate exercise routines.

Not only does exercise make it harder for cholesterol to stick to the walls of your arteries; it also reduces levels of bad cholesterol. Exercise causes your body to make more of the good, or HDL, cholesterol, which acts like a Roto-Rooter to sweep the bad, or LDL, cholesterol out of your bloodstream.

A third positive factor is that the heart, like any other muscle, gets bigger and stronger when used a lot. So a regular walking routine results in a stronger heart, one that can pump more blood with every beat, which means it doesn't have to work as hard to do its job.

Diabetes

We are in the midst of a diabetes epidemic in this country and we have nothing to blame but our modern lifestyles. If ever there was a lifestyle disease, type 2 diabetes is it. Type 2 diabetes is triggered by high-fat, high-carbohydrate (sugar and starch) diets, in conjunction with inactive living. That one-two punch describes too many of us and helps to explain why there are 17 million Americans with diabetes, up from just 10 million in 1990.

Even if we know that diabetes is a problem, many of us don't really understand the disease. Diabetes results when more glucose (sugar) is in the blood than the body can handle. The glucose comes from sugar we eat and from starches that the body easily converts to sugar. The body produces the hormone insulin to store as much as possible of the glucose in our muscle cells. The rest gets stored as fat. After awhile, however, our cells can't handle any more glucose and they start to resist the storing action, leaving the glucose to circulate in the blood. To compensate, the pancreas makes more insulin as a way of forcing that glucose out of the blood and into cells, but eventually the cells become too resistant to the insulin, the pancreas breaks down, and the body is left with dangerous levels of blood sugar.

Why dangerous? Because high levels of glucose damage artery walls, leading to the same blockages caused by too much cholesterol, with the same results: heart disease and stroke. That's why diabetes is a major factor in cardiovascular disease. And it is why *two out of every three diabetics will eventually die from heart disease or stroke.*

This is pretty alarming, but there is good news. Since this type of diabetes is a lifestyle disease, it is easily combated by lifestyle changes. Walking as little as three hours a week reduces your risk of diabetes by a whopping 58 percent! Follow my Walk Diet religiously, lay off the sweets, and you can be almost certain diabetes will never be a part of your life.

If you are one of the many women who discover my program after being diagnosed with diabetes, there is good news for you, too. Women with diabetes who walk a few miles per week lower their chance of developing cardiovascular disease by 40 percent. And they reduce their risk of dying from all causes by 39 percent! They can control their diabetes and lead normal lives. In fact, walking is such good medicine for diabetes that my program is being used in the national Look AHEAD (Action for Health in Diabetes) Study. This study, being carried out in sixteen centers around the United States, takes overweight people age fifty-five to seventy-five with type 2 diabetes and puts them on a program of exercise five times a week to reduce their level of heart attack and stroke. At the University of Pittsburgh's Look AHEAD Center, participants follow a program very similar to the one in this book.

If I could declare war on one disease, it would be diabetes. And I have just the troops to fight it: a legion of walkers, marching diabetes out of American homes, out of our children's lives, out of retirement centers. We could do it, too. Keep that thought in mind if you struggle through that last mile of walking for the day. Think, I'm marching diabetes out of my life.

Breast Cancer

Few words strike fear into a woman's heart like those two. Cancer is the second-leading killer in America, responsible for one of every four natural deaths, and breast cancer seems especially scary. But as with heart disease, exercise is particularly effective against breast cancer. Walking just two miles per week reduces your chance of breast cancer by 20 percent. Rev yourself up to spend at least four hours per week doing brisk exercise and you reduce your risk by 37 percent. Walking gives people protection against other cancers, too, especially colon and prostate cancer. We don't completely know why this is. My guess: the fact that walking keeps your weight down, the boost in immune function you get from moderate exercise, plus the "oil change" effect—by flushing all parts of your body with fresh blood and nutrients, walking helps keep waste products and toxins from accumulating.

Osteoporosis

By now, most women know that as they age, they are at risk for osteoporosis—decrease in bone mass. Twenty-eight million Americans have the disease, mostly older women. After age thirty-five, we women start to lose about 1 percent of our bone mass *every year*, and that number doubles after menopause. If this situation isn't held in check, simple falls result in broken hips, legs, and pelvises. Many fractures never heal. Spines slump and shorten. Your whole body *aches*.

We all know that we are supposed to take calcium supplements to prevent this (bones are largely composed of calcium), but few people realize that exercise is just as effective in maintaining bone density. Why? We think of bones much like we do brick or rock—as something hard, unyielding, and permanent. But that's only because we're used to seeing bones in a pork chop or a museum exhibit instead of as part of a living creature. Under your skin and muscle, your bones are very much alive. True, they are harder than the rest of you (good thing, too!), but they are more flexible than you'd imagine. They are also constantly rebuilding themselves.

In a way, it helps to think of bones as very hard muscle. Bones use calcium and

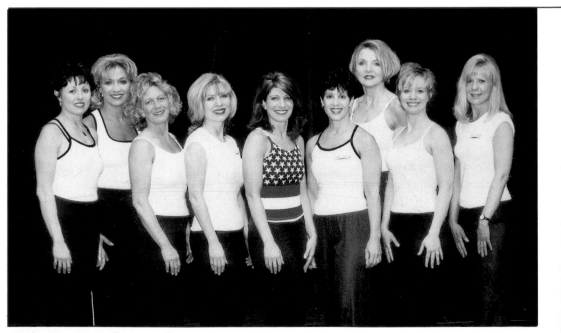

Coming soon to a mall near you!

other minerals as the "cement" to make them hard, while muscles are made of more flexible proteins, but they function similarly otherwise. The outer part of a bone is filled with blood vessels; bones become bigger and stronger when you exercise and break down when you don't, although the changes don't happen nearly as fast with bone as with muscle. Your muscles are attached to your bones, and the pulling of the muscles on the bones—the stress—signals your body to reinforce the bone. Aerobic exercise such as walking helps strengthen bones—especially in the lower half of the body—but strength training really does the trick, which is why training to develop upper-body strength is a key part of the Walk Diet.

Arthritis

Don't listen to people who tell you not to exercise too much as you age because it's hard on your joints. It's hard on your joints if you *don't* exercise. Like every other part of you, your joints were made to be used. That's what keeps them limber. Studies show that women who exercise regularly suffer much less joint pain than women who don't. They may still have arthritis; it just doesn't affect them as severely.

Immune System

Your immune system consists of special cells that zip around your body like little FBI agents, wiping out bad-guy cells (viruses, bacteria, and cancer cells) whenever they find them. If some bad-guy cells are able to hang around long enough to establish a colony, you get sick unless your immune cells can eliminate the colony. During exercise and for a few hours afterward, your body has more of these immune cells zipping through it. Because your heart is pumping more blood throughout your body, they circulate faster, too. This excellent system developed when most of our exercise involved chasing food or trying to avoid becoming food—situations when chances of injury and infection were high. This means you have little chance of catching a cold during or immediately after exercise—in other words, now's the time to wipe your three-year-old's nose!

Immune cells are another of the many systems that decline as we age, but once again, it's walking to the rescue! Active older women have as many immune cells as inactive women in their twenties.

Warning: Exercising to exhaustion creates just the opposite effect. Marathoners tend to get many colds after competing because they have very few immune cells left in their bodies. Basically, when you exercise extremely long and hard, your body panics and starts making extra fuel with the protein it normally uses to manufacture immune cells. So don't try to swim the English Channel—stick to walking!

Depression and Stress

Anytime I'm in a funk, the first thing I try to do is lace up my sneakers and walk it off. After a half hour of moving, more often than not I've forgotten whatever I was stewing over. I'm not alone in this. Lots of people know that the number-one difference in their mood at the end of the day is whether they've exercised or not. Many studies show regular exercise to be just as effective as drugs in treating mild depression. In fact, one study of older women whose depression was *not* helped by drugs found that half of them responded to ten weeks of exercise.

Why does exercise do this? Thank endorphins, for part of it. Exercise raises the level of these natural feel-good brain chemicals. It also burns off the adrenaline and other hormones created by stress that leave you ragged, sad, and sleepless. You can literally walk off stress! Knowing that exercise improves our looks and capabilities certainly helps our self-esteem, as well. But there sure seems to be more going on than this; sweets trigger endorphins, too, but they don't chase away the blues like a crisp autumn walk.

We'd like to think we're more complex than that. A bad mood or minor depression is the result of deep and intricate factors in our life, right? How could something as simple as a walk relieve it? But I suspect it is the other way around. You're in a funk because you haven't exercised, but you end up attributing it to whatever minor bumps you experienced in your day—you had an argument with your boss, or you were stuck in traffic for an hour. When you walk and have that good feeling *inside* that exercise gives you, you shake off the little things.

In reality, we aren't all that complicated, and I think that's a wonderful thing. The formula for a happy life is pretty darned simple: active body, active mind, active spirit, active social life. The challenge stems from how easy it has become to let one, two, or more of these things slip away from us.

If I were you, I wouldn't worry so much about the *why* part of it. Exercise makes you feel good and allows you to shake off stress like water droplets. Don't think about it too hard; just do it.

Alzheimer's Disease and Memory Loss

I know, it seems like once you turn thirty, every part of your body starts getting larger on its own, but there is actually one part that starts to shrink at that age. Unfortunately, it's your brain! Scientists have long known that our brains lose cells as we age and that this contributes to the diseases we associate with mental decline: Alzheimer's disease, Huntington's disease, and plain old memory loss. Scientists also know that fit people are less likely to suffer mental decline with age. Now they think they've figured out why: high blood-sugar levels are responsible for the brain shrinkage. Diabetic and obese people are the ones most likely to have high blood-sugar levels, and exercise is the best way to keep off the pounds and regulate blood-sugar levels. (Muscle literally absorbs sugar for energy.) Studies show that older adults can even reverse mental decline by starting to exercise.

Hey, this even works for rats. Rats forced to play and exercise had 25 percent more synapses in their brains than rats forced to take it easy. So exercise, unless you fancy life as a rat couch potato!

Other Conditions

Exercise has a positive effect on almost any physical condition you can think of—it really is a miracle—but some of the most notable ones are asthma, emphysema, chronic back pain, ulcers, indigestion, and irritable bowel syndrome. If you have a condition I haven't mentioned and are wondering whether exercise will alleviate it, ask your doctor.

The Big Kahuna

I couldn't sum it up better than this: Women who are active reduce their risk of premature death from all causes by 55 percent. Love life? Keep walking!

4. Before You Begin

Notice how blessedly short this chapter is! One of the reasons people like my program is because they can get started so quickly. The basic moves can be learned in a matter of seconds. I'll demonstrate them all in the following chapters. Other than that, the only things you need to consider are what you wear and whether you have any health conditions that will be affected.

Walking is naturally safe. If this was a running book, I'd have to spend a lot of time teaching you how not to hurt yourself. Running produces four times as much force on the feet and joints, which is why almost everyone who runs long enough suffers foot, ankle, or knee problems. This doesn't happen to walkers. Walking is, in fact, one of the very safest forms of exercise. Still, there are a few no-nos to be avoided when choosing attire, using weights, or walking through illness, so read on. Pay attention to a few basic rules and you will walk healthy and safe for your entire life.

GEAR

As I said earlier, with my program you can walk in your birthday suit if you want. You are in your own living room. No one is around. . . . Do what you want! The one place you can't show any skin, however, is your feet. A sure way to promote foot injuries is to walk many miles barefoot. To avoid that, I'm going to give you some strong advice on footwear. Most of you probably want to wear a bit more than just shoes, so I cover all the other considerations you need to make, too, from socks and sweats to the tools that can help you get your upper body firm and strong.

Shoes

You'd be amazed what people try to walk in. They walk in plastic sneakers, they walk in old sneakers, they walk in shoes with no support, and they even walk in sandals! They think, I'm just walking, so what could it matter?

Well, it does matter—a lot. Think about it: All your weight is coming down on one tiny arch two thousand times for every mile you walk. An active person's feet will hit the ground ten thousand times a day! Try thumping your hand with a book ten thousand times and see if padding might make a difference.

Here is one of the few times in life when shopping will actually save you money. Before you start walking, go out and get yourself the set of walking shoes that is absolutely perfect for you. That doesn't mean the sneakers on sale for $19.95. They are cheap for a reason. Cheap shoes generally have cheap rubber treads, which wear out, or inferior midsoles, which don't provide much shock absorption and break down quickly, leaving you with no arch support. Don't skimp on shoes! You are more likely to quit an exercise program if your arches ache and you develop blisters every time you work out.

When you spend the forty or fifty dollars for quality sneakers or walking shoes, you get materials that won't degrade in a few months, and you get an arch and padding that suit your activity. Good running shoes or cross-trainers are fine for walking, but the cushioning is actually a bit different in a true walking shoe because your heel and pad hit the ground at a different angle. If your sneakers work well for you, stick with them. If you suffer any pain during or after walking, try true walking shoes.

The money-saving part comes from the fact that you won't be making any trips to the doctor for foot pain, and because if well-fitting shoes keep you exercising more, then you get the health and weight-loss benefits and make fewer trips to the doctor for *all* reasons. Do you really need more convincing? Get out there and shop!

Here's what you want to look for: good cushioning for your heels and toes, a tight fit that supports your instep but leaves wiggle room for your toes, quality construction, and breathable upper materials (mesh or leather). The better brands now offer versions customized to your particular arch. People with flat arches need extra arch support to help spread the force of each impact, while people with high arches tend to have feet that roll out slightly upon impact, putting extra stress on the outside of the ankle.

And now a word about shoe size. Many women try to jam their feet into sneakers a size too small because they think smaller feet are somehow more attractive. Come on, Cinderella, put away that size six and get a shoe that fits! Small shoes cause pain and toe blisters. Shoes that are too roomy also cause blisters because they slide. And shoes designed for men won't fit right, either: Men's feet tend to be wider at the heel and narrower at the toe. Get yourself fitted professionally. You'll thank yourself later.

Once you have the perfect pair of shoes, use them like crazy and then get new ones once a year. Even the best shoes wear down after heavy use, at which point they won't function much better than cheap ones.

There are many good walking shoes on the market, but the following models are recommended by the American Academy of Podiatry Sports Medicine (www.aapsm.org) specifically for walking:

Brooks WT Leather Addiction
Rockport World Tour
Rockport Prowalker DMX
New Balance 840 Series
New Balance 810 Series
Asics Tech Walker

You can also find shoes with an undercarriage that allows them to function like walking shoes but a stylish chassis that makes them look like office shoes. Ask your favorite shoe store for some recommendations.

Socks

Even people who drop eighty dollars for a top pair of athletic shoes sometimes pay no attention to socks. They figure a sock is a sock, so they pull on their cotton crews and start walking. But all socks are not created equal. And even the conventional wisdom you often hear from doctors or magazines can be quite wrong.

For instance, cotton socks are best because they breathe better than polyester, right? Wrong. It's true that early polyester fabrics tended to trap moisture, but modern acrylic ones can be designed to wick away moisture at a rate that no cotton sock can match. Cotton is extremely absorbent, which means that at first it does a great job of removing sweat from your foot. (The drier the foot, the more comfortable you'll be.) Cotton just keeps on absorbing sweat, however, so soon you have a wet sock around you. Acrylic socks, on the other hand, can strike a nice balance between absorbing and repelling moisture. They take the moisture off your foot and transfer it to the shoe, or to the top of the sock. If your shoe breathes well, the moisture will evaporate and your foot can stay dry indefinitely. Overall, cotton is three times more absorbent than acrylic and fourteen times more so than CoolMax, a special fabric designed with extra space between the fibers to wick away sweat and keep you cool and dry. Cotton and wool socks also tend to stretch and bunch more than acrylic, making them more uncomfortable as they wear.

The U.S. Army is especially interested in socks. Troops suffer horrendous blister problems from their months of marching and training in boots. In recent years, the problem got so bad that the army commissioned studies comparing their traditional cotton/wool socks with acrylic and CoolMax socks. The results showed such a reduction in blisters from the synthetic socks that the army has now switched.

Depending on your feet and your walking program, you may be just fine in your cotton socks. If you have no problems, then there's no reason to switch. If you do have discomfort, get a sock that is designed to wick away moisture and that also has plenty of padding. Then you will have no blister problems. If you walk indoors and tend to get warm, choose CoolMax or another fabric designed to keep your feet cool and comfortable.

Want to know another mistake almost everybody makes? They spend plenty of time choosing just the right shoe, then pick up their socks as an afterthought on the way out of the store. Socks can be quite different from one another, and this can affect your whole shoe size. Pick out your socks *first*; then try on shoes while wearing the socks they'll be paired with. The eighteen-year-old clerk may look at you funny, but you are going to be spending a lot less time with him than you are with your own feet.

Clothing

This is where the beauty of indoor walking shines through! Other than shoes and socks, your clothing needs are incredibly simple and flexible. No bundling up against the cold or rain. No balancing warmth or water protection against breathability. Just put on your shorts and T-shirt and away you go. If you keep your house cool, you can wear sweats instead, but chances are you'll warm up fast, so try shorts or tights first.

One piece of clothing you may want to consider is a sports bra. These are essential for pregnant women, but most other women I know also prefer them while exercising. They reduce stress on your back, minimize bouncing, and maximize comfort. There are a dazzling number of models and styles, so try out different kinds before choosing.

Hand Weights

Holding small weights—just one or two pounds—while you walk is the easiest way to increase your calorie burning and muscle toning. You don't do anything differently than during a normal walk, and they are light enough that you hardly notice the difference. But the difference is there: Your upper-body muscles are working harder every second of the walk, making this a great way to squeeze maximum calorie burn into a short time.

I am not a fan of dumbbells. The fist you make when you grip them, and the way they stick out awkwardly on either side of your hand, means that you can't walk normally while carrying them. You have to hold your arms out unnaturally, which increases your chance of pulling muscles in your arms, shoulders, and back. Soft weighted balls or weighted gloves that slide right on your hands are much better choices for normal arm action. As a bonus, the squishy balls hurt much less when they get dropped on your toes, and the gloves don't get dropped at all! If you don't want to spend any money on weights, you can find objects around your house that weigh a pound or two (such as filled plastic water bottles—eight- to sixteen-ounce capacity) and fit comfortably in your hand.

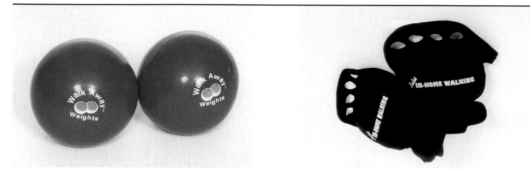

Weighted balls or gloves are the easiest way to tone your arms and back without risking injury.

Start off with one- or two-pound weights so you don't strain yourself. As you get stronger and want to continue challenging your larger muscles, you can increase the weight to a maximum of three pounds.

Never lock your joints when using weights. Keep your arms bent so the pressure is on the muscles, not the fragile joints. I like to hold the weights by my sides and walk normally, then hold them over my head for a count of ten, and then bring them back to my sides. See my demonstration on page 48 for more specific instructions.

Warning: Many people assume that because light hand weights are such a good idea, they can double their fat blasting by strapping on ankle weights, too. Bad idea! Your arms swing freely while walking and don't impact anything. Your legs, on the other hand, hit the floor with every step. Ankle weights make you walk like a moose. They throw off your natural stride and cause every impact with the floor to be a little off. The result? Lots and lots of twisted ankles—or worse. Tendonitis can be caused or aggravated by ankle weights. Your knees suffer from the extra strain, too. You also may have noticed that your back muscles are connected to your legs. Every step pulls on the muscles in your back, so if you want to throw out your back, then by all means wear ankle weights while you walk.

Ab Belt

At first, an ab belt doesn't look like much: How could a little piece of nylon and rubber you wear around your waist improve your fitness? You'll be surprised. In fact, an ab belt helps you burn calories the whole time you are wearing it, not just when you work out. As soon as you strap it on, you feel a light pressure against your abdomen. That pressure forces your muscles to work a little, and working means burning calories, toning, and weight loss.

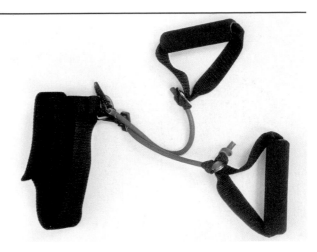

An ab belt with rubber resistance cords tones not only your abs but your entire upper body.

Of course, the real benefits kick in when you work out with the belt. The hand straps are on rubber cords, which resist as you try to pull them away from your body. This resistance requires you to work harder. Bingo: strength training, upper-body toning, and an all-over workout just by swinging your arms. What a perfect complement to my failproof walking plan! You can even get different cords to adjust the resistance level.

In my belt routines, I take the toning benefits a step further by incorporating various arm stretches. You can teach yourself by following my instructions on page 50. You'll have it down in about two minutes. Ab belts are available at most sporting goods or discount stores.

Stretch Band

A stretch band is like having the world's smallest fitness center in your gym bag. It's just a ten-dollar strip of plastic, but it can work all the muscles in your arms, back, chest, and shoulders. Not only that, but because the stretch band is so flexible, you can constantly change the angle at which you engage your muscles, which helps ensure that every little bit of them gets involved. You can also increase the stretch band's power by shortening your grip on the band, so it's like a whole set of weights in one. (For this reason, if you don't want to spend much money on equipment, you can get a stretch band and use it for all your strength training; just substitute it for the

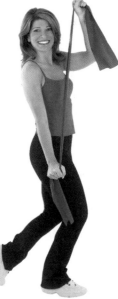

Here I am with my Stretchie. People love the variety of ways they can use it!

weights or belt anytime they are recommended.) Potential ways to use the stretch band are as unlimited as your imagination. See my demonstrations on page 51 for some ideas; then see what else you can come up with. You can order a stretch band at my Web site or pick one up at your nearest discount store.

Pedometer

If you prefer unstructured exercise to structured exercise, consider getting a pedometer. The pedometer, or step counter, is a neat little device that clips onto your sneakers and counts every time your foot hits the floor. At the end of the day, you can see how many steps you've taken. If you are following the miles on the walking program, this isn't really necessary, but some people like to get their walking in by increasing the number of steps they take while going about a normal day. There are many ways to do this. Walk around the block at lunch, always choose steps instead of elevators, park once in town and walk to all your errands, or even take a hike. A pedometer will tell you just how much exercise you're getting.

You may be surprised by the results. I was! To get optimum health and weight-loss benefits, you need to approach 10,000 steps per day (instead of the 3,000 the average adult gets). That means you're covering about five miles. (In my program, half of that is in scheduled walks and the other half comes through your normal activities.) People have mistaken me for the Energizer Bunny; I go, go, go all the time. So I was pretty sure that I covered 10,000 steps, no problem. I mean, I'm "Walk Girl!" On a day when I had no fitness activities scheduled, I clipped on a pedometer and away I went: to the studio, around the studio, back home, upstairs, downstairs, back out, in again. By the time I hit the bed that night and took off my counter, I was shocked. Know what my count was? Only 6,755!

That pedometer was a swift kick in the rear. Now I try to get in 10,000 steps every day. And that should be your goal, too, if you go the step-counting route. Don't aim for 10,000 right away, however. That would be like starting off doing three miles of walking every day without ever having done one mile. Wear the step counter for a few days before you begin exercising in order to get your average steps per day. Then add 500 steps to that number each day until you hit 10,000. Don't fool yourself; you'll need to schedule some walks to hit 10,000—unless you are a city mailman!

Some pedometers talk, telling you how many steps you've done and how many you have left to reach your goal. That's a nice feature, because you don't need to stop your walks to keep checking it. A range of pedometers is available at most discount and sporting goods stores.

Heart-Rate Monitor

I haven't discussed heart rate in this book because I wanted to keep things simple, but some people like to tailor their exercise to their heart rate. To do this, you first must determine your maximum heart rate—the absolute fastest your heart can beat—by subtracting your age from 220 (because hearts can't go as fast as they age). If you are fifty, your maximum heart rate is $220 - 50 = 170$. You are in the aerobic zone, burning fat, whenever your heart is beating at 60 to 80 percent of maximum rate. Below 60 percent, you aren't working hard enough to need to burn fat; above 80 percent, your heart can't pump enough oxygen to your muscles and you stop burning fat. The simple way to monitor this is to do the "talk test." If you can gab all you want without stopping, you haven't hit 60 percent of maximum heart rate and aren't getting the health benefits. If you are breathing deeply and can get out a few short sentences, you are in the aerobic zone. If you are gasping for breath and can manage only a few words, you are in the anaerobic zone and burning sugar.

The catch: As you get more fit, your heart doesn't have to work as hard to do the same workout. Maybe a one-mile walk got your heart up to 70 percent when you started, but now it only gets you to 50 percent. You need to do that second mile (or a faster first mile) to get the cardiovascular benefits and to burn fat. If using heart rate as a guide interests you, a heart-rate monitor removes the guesswork. You can order one from my Web site or pick one up at a discount or sporting goods store.

HEALTH CONDITIONS

Walking is for *everyone*—fit and unfit, old and young, male and female. So often I hear from people who want to start walking but think they can't because of a particular health condition. In almost all these cases, the truth is that walking is one of the best things they can do for their health concerns. Short of a coma, few health conditions preclude walking. There are a few, however, where it pays to be safe, so hear me loud and clear: *If you have health concerns of any kind, check with your physician before beginning this or any other fitness program.* Your doctor will be thrilled to hear you're considering a fitness program and will help you get started safely and painlessly. To anticipate what your doctor might tell you, you can scan through this section to find the health condition that concerns you and learn some of the facts. You'll probably find that what you thought was a problem keeping you out of the game permanently will turn out to be nothing more than a brief stint on the sidelines.

Heart Disease

A lot of heart attacks occur during exercise, right? Well, would you believe only 5 percent, and that almost all of those occur in high-risk individuals engaged in *strenuous* exercise like snow shoveling? If you are a normal fifty-year-old, your chance of having a heart attack during strenuous exercise is one in a million—literally! Your chance of having one while walking is no higher than of having one while sleeping. If you have experienced problems with your ticker, you need to get on a walking program right away—but a *gradual* one. Few things can better restore your health. Stay away from harder exercises, which can put you at risk. Consider using a heart monitor to help you stay in the exercise zone that best combines safety with health improvement. Your physician can help design a program that matches your current abilities. If you haven't had any heart problems, walking will help ensure that you never will.

High Blood Pressure

High blood pressure often leads to heart problems or stroke, and people suffering from it are at more risk when they exercise hard. Blood pressure goes up during exercise. Experts recommend that if your blood pressure is higher than 160/100 mm Hg, you do something about it before hitting the weights or the StairMaster. Check with your physician. One of the things likely to be recommended to you is *walking*.

Diabetes

The big issue for diabetics is blood-sugar level. It is important to keep this nice and even, but exercise tends to deplete blood sugar as the sugar gets burned for fuel. Over the long term, exercise is essential to keep your body metabolizing blood sugar, but you should monitor your blood-sugar level closely before and after exercise. If you use insulin, it may be best to take a shot before exercising. Drink lots of water, too. Again, your doctor will know exactly what level of walking matches your condition and abilities.

Arthritis

If you have arthritis or joint pain in your hips, knees, or ankles, you need to walk a fine line between too much and too little exercise. During a flare-up, it is probably best to put as little pressure on your legs as possible. The rest of the time, gentle walking—and I mean *gentle*—is one of the best ways to prevent stiffness and keep joint pain to a minimum.

Dizziness or Fainting

If you suffer from either of these on a regular basis, you have a deeper underlying problem. See your doctor right away.

WARM UP AND COOL DOWN

Warming up at the beginning of your walk and cooling down at the end not only prevent injury but also improve your performance. Begin each walk with a few minutes of gradual pacing to get fluid flowing into muscles and joints and to heat up your muscles. Warm muscle is more pliable, meaning you're less likely to pull a muscle. It also can absorb more oxygen and fuel. You've probably had that classic experience of launching immediately into some form of exercise and finding yourself panting after only five minutes. You may have thought you were out of energy, but you weren't; your cold muscles just couldn't get enough oxygen. So your lungs were working harder to try to compensate, and without oxygen, your muscles were burning only sugar, not fat. Let yourself warm up before exercising and you will get injured less, perform better, burn more fat, and flush away lactic acid more quickly, meaning less soreness. Cooling down at the end of your workout by pacing slowly until your heart rate and breathing are back to normal also helps remove lactic acid and prevents a situation where your muscles aren't using new blood anymore but your heart is still forcing extra through your arteries.

PART II

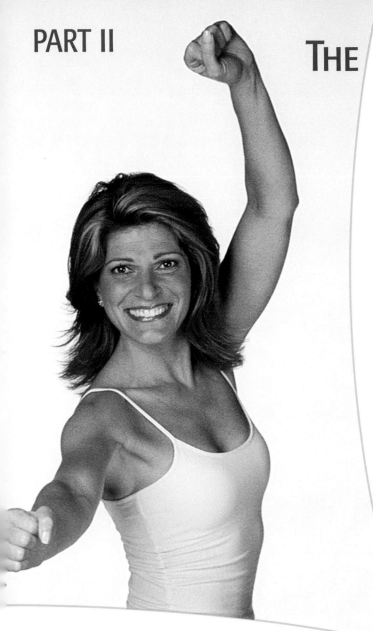

THE
EXERCISES

WALKING IS THE BEST POSSIBLE EXERCISE.
HABITUATE YOURSELF TO WALK VERY FAR.

—— THOMAS JEFFERSON

5. Basic Walking Moves

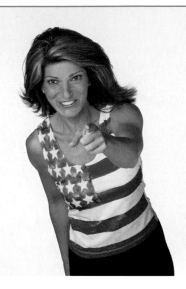

There are four basic steps that I work into all my walks. Mixing these steps into your routine ensures that you engage as many muscles as possible. It also keeps you energized! The first step is about as basic as it gets.

WALK IN PLACE

Begin each workout by walking as you normally do. You know how to walk, but you can check my form for pointers. My foot is raised perhaps six inches off the ground, and my opposite arm swings forward at the same time. It's essential to have good upright posture while walking—or doing anything else, for that matter! Your abdominal muscles should be tight and your shoulder blades retracted to get that beautiful spinal alignment that prevents sore backs. One thing you'll find about walking in place is that you end up lifting your knees higher than if you're walking forward.

Choose your pace based on your abilities and goals. However long or fast you intend to go, begin each walk with several minutes of gentle warm-up. This is vitally important in order to get your blood pumping through your muscles and fluid lubricating your joints. Warming up not only prevents injuries but also allows your muscles to perform at a higher level without tiring, so it will make you a better, stronger walker.

Once you feel your heart starting to pick up, increase your pace. Pump your arms to get your upper body involved and to boost the calorie burn. (This also helps your balance.) The right pace for you is whatever keeps you in that middle rate of exertion, where you can pass the "talk test"—you aren't gasping, can talk if necessary, but your lungs are working harder than normal. I usually

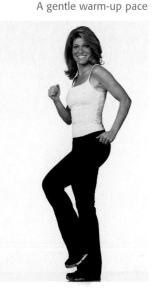

A gentle warm-up pace

try to get people walking at about two steps per second, which works out to about a fifteen-minute mile. That's pretty fast! It may be too brisk for you at first, but you'll work up to it in no time.

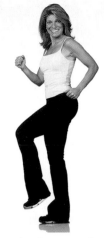

A good midwalk pace, with the foot nice and high for extra calorie burn

SIDE STEPS

After a few minutes of walking in place, you are ready to mix in some side steps. These are a great way to work your thighs and backside to get that nicely sculpted core. The pace is ever so slightly slower than walking in place, because the motion takes longer.

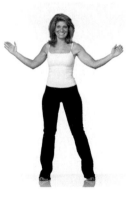 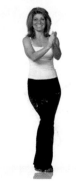 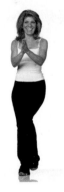

1. STEP TO YOUR LEFT with your left foot, continuing to face forward. Your arm action should mirror your legs: Spread them wide as you step.

2. BRING YOUR RIGHT foot together with your left. Bring your hands together at the same time.

3. STEP BACK TO YOUR RIGHT with your right foot, spreading your arms again.

4. BRING YOUR LEFT FOOT together with your right foot. Bring your hands together at the same time.

Repeat this four-step move ten times; then return to walking in place for another minute or two, then do another ten side steps. Now you are beginning to see why walking in place allows you to do things you could never do on an outdoor walk! Once you are comfortable with these two basic steps, you are ready to work the third step into your routine.

KICKS

Kicks give the quadriceps (the front thigh muscles) and backside a little extra workout. The four-step move is similar to that for side steps.

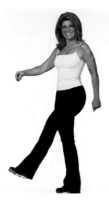 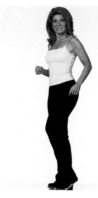 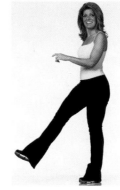 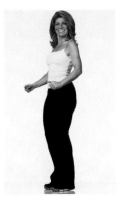

1. KICK YOUR LEFT LEG forward at a comfortable distance.

2. BRING YOUR FOOT BACK to the ground.

3. KICK YOUR RIGHT LEG forward at a comfortable distance.

4. BRING YOUR FOOT BACK to the ground.

The kick shouldn't break you out of your pace. You aren't trying to pull a Bruce Lee move on anybody. Also make sure you don't lean back when kicking; if you lean back, you won't get the full muscle benefit. Repeat this four-step move ten times; then return to walking in place. Continue to mix in one or two minutes of walking in place with ten counts of side steps and kicks (always returning to walking in place in between). Once you are comfortable with these three basic steps, you are ready to work the fourth step into your routine.

KNEE LIFTS

The knee lift gives you the benefits of walking and crunches at the same time. Bringing your legs up with every step really works the abs and quads. The four-step motion is identical to that of the kicks, except you lift your knee up instead of kicking your foot out.

Repeat this four-step move ten times; then return to walking in place. You now have the four basic moves down and should mix them all into your routines.

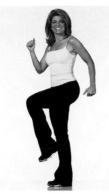
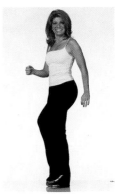

1. LIFT YOUR LEFT KNEE until it is nearly horizontal.

2. BRING IT BACK DOWN.

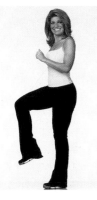
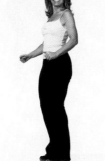
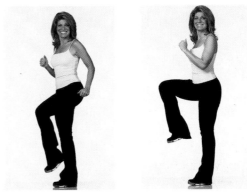

3. LIFT YOUR RIGHT KNEE until it is nearly horizontal.

4. BRING IT BACK DOWN.

You can adjust the height of the knee lift depending on your abilities. Note the less strenuous lift in the first picture and then the perfectly horizontal lift in the second—yeah, girl!

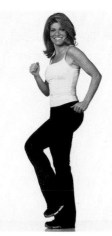

COOL DOWN

An essential part of healthy walking is the cool-down period at the end. During the last few minutes of your walk, reduce your intensity until you are back to that gentle warm-up pace. This allows you to bring your heartbeat back to its regular rate in a gradual fashion, preventing the situation where your muscles have stopped working but your heart is still pounding in your chest.

A nice relaxed cool-down stride

STRETCHES

No matter what my routine, I always end it with some gentle stretches to keep my muscles loose and pliant for my next workout. Some people stretch before a workout, but I don't like the feeling of stretching cold muscle. It feels best to me to warm up your muscles with gentle walking, and save the stretch until the end of your walk.

Why stretch at the end? Because, while physical activity is vital for keeping your body young and healthy, it does put stress on your muscles. With walking, most of that stress is concentrated in the calves, thighs, and lower back. After activity, these muscles tend to tighten and shorten. Stretching at the end keeps them loose and also keeps them *long*, meaning you get more of that ballerina look even when you're not exercising.

It only takes a minute or two to go through my stretch routine, but it makes all the difference in how you'll feel throughout the day!

1. Overhead Stretch

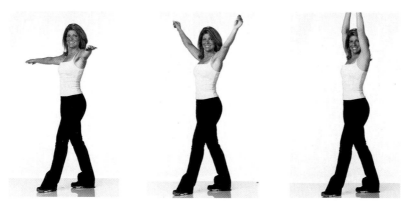

STARTING WITH YOUR ARMS DOWN AT YOUR SIDES, smoothly raise them out to the sides, up, and overhead. Inhale as you raise them. Hold them overhead for a few seconds; then smoothly lower them back to your sides, exhaling on the way down. Repeat three times.

2. Calf Stretch

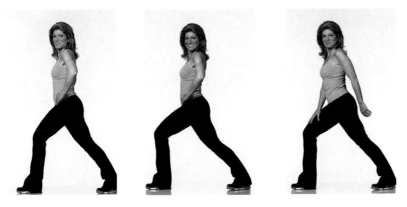

1. TURN TO YOUR RIGHT SIDE, step forward with your right foot, and plant your left heel solidly behind you. Keep your toes pointing directly forward.

2. SCOOT YOUR LEFT HEEL BACK, keeping it against the ground, until you feel the stretch in your left calf. Check your alignment. You want a straight back in order to give you the long spine that helps the stretch.

3. PLACING YOUR RIGHT HAND ON YOUR RIGHT THIGH to support your back, move your hips forward. You'll feel the pull on your calf and lower back. Then see how far forward you can lean. Don't overdo it, but try to give yourself a nice stretch for a few seconds. Then stand back up and repeat on the other side.

3. Quad Stretch

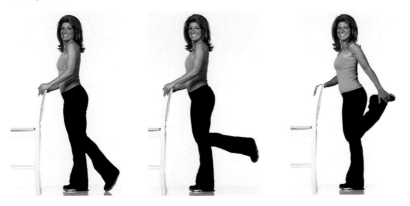

1. HOLD THE BACK OF A CHAIR WITH YOUR HANDS. Your hips should be facing forward and your back should be straight. Don't slouch.

2. LIFT YOUR LEFT FOOT STRAIGHT UP BEHIND YOU.

3. GRAB YOUR LEFT FOOT WITH YOUR LEFT HAND and help lift it up toward your backside. You'll feel the stretch in your quadricep (the front of your thigh). Only go as far as is comfortable. Hold the position for a few seconds; then lower your foot and repeat on the other side.

4. Hamstring Stretch

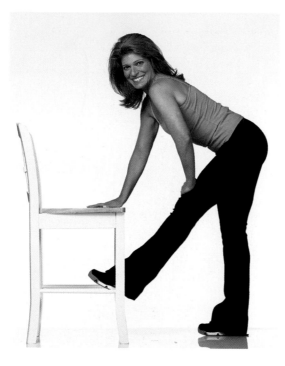

USING A CHAIR WITH A LOWER RUNG (about a foot off the ground), prop your left foot on the chair. Lean forward, putting your left hand on your left thigh and your right hand on the chair seat for support. Keep your leg and back as straight as possible. You'll feel the stretch in your hamstring (the back of your thigh). Hold the position for a few seconds; then stand back up and repeat on the other side.

5. Back Stretch

FACE THE FRONT OF A CHAIR, standing about two feet away. Grab the back of the chair and lean forward until your arms and back are parallel to the ground. You'll feel the stretch in your lower back. Hold the position for several seconds; then straighten up.

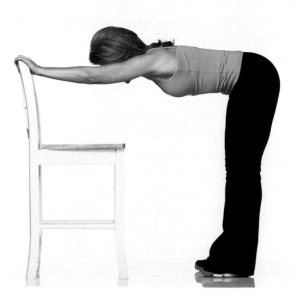

6. Strength-Training Moves

Beginning with Week 3 of your program (or right away if you are an experienced walker), you should work strength training into your routine. Other chapters of this book tell you about all the fat-burning, muscle-sculpting, bone-strengthening benefits you get from it. I've found that most walkers like to keep their routines interesting by mixing a variety of strength-training equipment into their walks, so I demonstrate three different kinds here and recommend the three at various points in the six-week Walk Diet. But you are free to use all three, to choose whatever equipment appeals to you most and stick with that, or to use something else you already have at home.

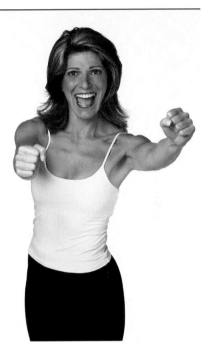

Once you are comfortable with these moves, as well as the basic steps, you can start to customize your own walking routines. Everyone has different needs, and there is no right or wrong way to work out; it all depends on your stamina, size, and goals. If you want to concentrate on firming your middle, you should mix in a lot of ab belt or stretch band moves, as well as knee lifts. If thighs are your issue, then lots of side steps while squatting slightly will be just the ticket. Whatever moves you choose, make sure you switch to something different every couple of minutes to work a variety of muscles and keep yourself interested.

WEIGHTED BALLS

These moves work well with any sort of hand weight, though I find weighted balls or gloves the easiest and safest. Whatever distance you walk, use the weights for about half the time and walk normally the other half.

To get comfortable with the weights, hold them in your hands in front of you as you pump your arms and go through your normal routine using the four basic walking steps. Just bringing this extra weight along makes your whole body work harder. Even if you feel you aren't ready for the strength-training moves, simply doing this will boost your calorie burn and firm your upper body beautifully.

1. Overhead Lift

1. HOLD THE WEIGHTS IN FRONT OF YOU and pump your arms normally as you walk.
2. RAISE THE WEIGHTS straight over your head for two steps.
3. BRING THE WEIGHTS BACK DOWN for two steps.

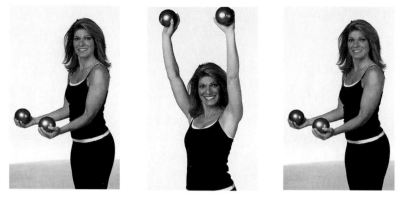

Repeat this move ten times. Then return to walking in place. Once you get used to this, you can increase the time you hold the weights over your head, up to ten steps. Make sure you always bring them back down for an equal period. Vary this amount as needed to keep you engaged. Or combine the overhead lift with the side reach.

2. Side Reach

Here you can see the weighted gloves I sometimes use. The exercise works the same way with balls or other hand weights.

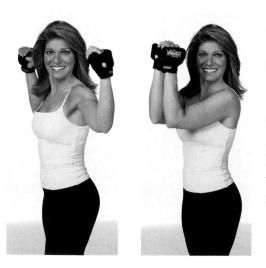

1. WHILE WALKING IN PLACE, spread your hands out to your sides and hold for two steps.
2. BRING YOUR HANDS TOGETHER in front of you for two steps.

Repeat this move ten times. Then return to walking in place. As with the previous move, you can vary the time you hold your hands out, up to ten steps. Always remember to return to walking in place for at least a minute between moves.

3. Bicep Curl

This classic arm-strengthening exercise will really make you feel like a weight lifter!

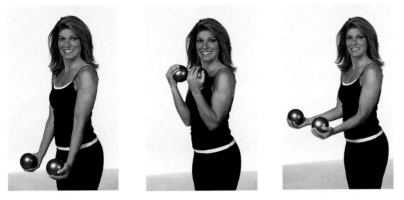

1. AS YOU WALK, hold the weights down at your waist.

2. BRING THEM UP toward your chest and hold them there for two steps.

3. DROP THEM BACK down for two steps.

Repeat this move ten times. Then return to walking in place before beginning your next move.

QUICK TIPS

- Try alternating your hands with the weight moves: one up and one down with the bicep curl, for example, then switching back and forth.
- Holding your hands straight out in front of you at arm's reach, instead of over your head, increases the workout for your back muscles.

AB BELT

Simply having an ab belt around your waist, pushing on your muscles, forces your muscles to push back. Bingo: waistline whittling! Attaching rubber cords to the belt and using it to work your arms sends the upper-body benefits sky-high. Abdominal muscles, biceps, triceps, deltoids, and back muscles all kick in. As with the other strength-training aids, use the ab belt for about half of your walk.

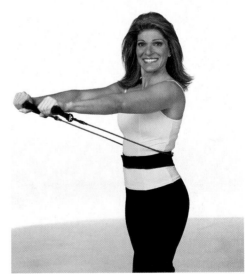

Note the proper way to attach the belt. The cords should be connected to the belt at your back.

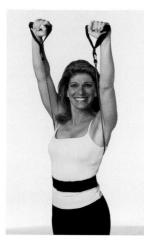

1. Overhead Lift

BEGIN BY HOLDING THE HANDLES AT YOUR WAIST; then slowly raise the handles straight over your head. The farther you reach, the stronger the resistance becomes. Hold the handles over your head for ten steps; then slowly bring them back down to your sides for ten steps.

Repeat ten times. Then return to regular walking before beginning your next move.

2. Side Reach

BEGINNING WITH THE HANDLES AT YOUR WAIST, stretch your arms straight out to your sides for two steps; then bring them back to your waist for two steps.

Repeat ten times. Then return to regular walking before beginning your next move.

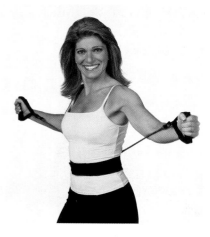

3. Front Reach

BEGINNING WITH THE HANDLES AT YOUR WAIST, stretch your arms straight out in front of you for two steps; then bring them back to your waist for two steps.

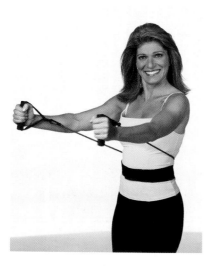

Repeat ten times. Then return to regular walking before beginning your next move.

When not being used, the handles can be tucked into the belt so they don't get in your way. As you get comfortable with the belt, you can find a mixture of overhead lifts, side reaches, front reaches, other moves, and regular walking that works well for you. You can do the belt moves with any of the four basic walking steps.

• Try combining the three basic belt moves in one rolling sequence: overhead, waist, sides, waist, front, waist.
• Throwing punches across your body (one arm at a time) with the handles engages the muscles at many different angles. And it's fun!

STRETCH BAND

A stretch band is as versatile a tool as you can imagine. By resisting you as you stretch it apart, it functions like weights (weights are just extra resistance against muscle), and it can roll up in your pocket and go anywhere with you. I love thinking up new ways to use the stretch band, but here are the basic moves to get you started. As with the other strength-training aids, use the stretch band for about half of your walk.

1. Front Reach

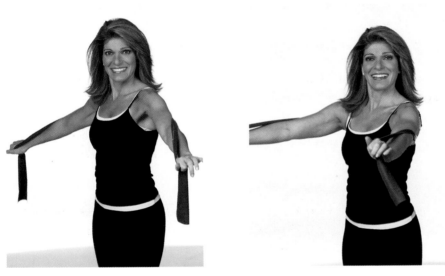

1. WRAP THE BAND AROUND YOUR BACK behind the shoulder blades.
2. REACH OUT STRAIGHT IN FRONT of you for two steps. Then let the band pull your hands back for two steps.

Feel the resistance. When you reach out, the band should pull back against you, but not so much that you have to struggle to get your hands forward. To increase the resistance, move your hands closer to the middle of the band. To reduce it, move them toward the ends. Repeat this move ten times, varying the angle of your arms slightly to work all parts of the muscle; then return to regular walking before beginning the next move.

2. Upward Reach

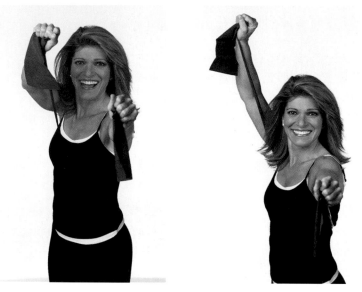

1. WRAP THE BAND AROUND YOUR BACK behind the shoulder blades.
2. REACH UP, PUSHING FORWARD just enough to keep the band from slipping up your back. Hold for two steps; then let the band pull your hands back for two steps.

Repeat ten times. Then return to regular walking before beginning your next move.

3. Diagonal Pull

I love moves like this one because they work the two sides of your body in different ways at the same time. Just remember to switch sides to keep yourself in balance!

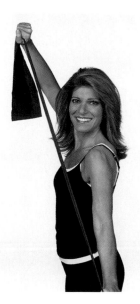

RAISE THE STRETCH BAND OVERHEAD with your right hand while you push it toward the ground with your left hand. Hold for two steps; then release the tension for two steps.

Repeat ten times; then switch and raise your left arm while lowering your right one ten times. Then return to regular walking before beginning your next move.

4. Backward Reach

Here is a great way to engage muscles in the chest, arms, and shoulders that rarely get worked.

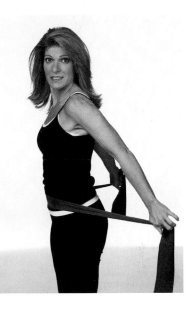

WRAP THE BAND ACROSS YOUR ABDOMEN and extend both arms behind you as far as possible. Hold for two steps; then release the tension for two steps.

Repeat ten times. Then return to regular walking before beginning your next move.

QUICK TIPS

- Try holding any of these moves for four steps instead of two. Notice any difference in the workout?
- For variety, try a "butterfly wing" move: Wrap the band around your back, reach out to your sides, and then, keeping your arms extended, bring them together in front of you for two steps before bringing them back to your sides for two steps.

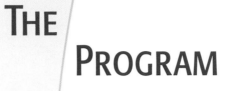

PART III

THE
PROGRAM

HAPPILY MAY I WALK.
MAY IT BE BEAUTIFUL BEFORE ME.
MAY IT BE BEAUTIFUL BEHIND ME.
MAY IT BE BEAUTIFUL BELOW ME.
MAY IT BE BEAUTIFUL ABOVE ME.
MAY IT BE BEAUTIFUL ALL AROUND ME.
IN BEAUTY IT IS FINISHED.

— NAVAHO NIGHT CHANT

7. The Walk Diet

If this was a typical weight-loss book, it would ask you to do one of two things right now: It would ask you either to take a long look at your diet and make some drastic changes or to take a long, hard look at yourself to determine why you're out of shape and what major personality flaw you can alter to improve your self-esteem.

Lucky for you, this is the *Walk Away the Pounds* fitness plan! In my twenty-five years of helping people get in shape, I've learned a few things, and one is that making drastic changes right off the bat backfires. It's just too hard. Another thing I've learned is that too much self-absorption doesn't lead to anything except more self-absorption! So save the "why" questions for later; once you've started exercising, you'll find that a lot of those questions just evaporate anyway—and the ones that are still there are a lot easier to think about. It's like those times you lie awake at three o'clock in the morning, obsessing over some minor problem. That headache that you were sure was brain cancer in the middle of the night turns out at breakfast to have been . . . well, a headache. The same applies to worrying about self-esteem when you're down. Don't bother; you won't see yourself realistically. Things are a lot better than you think.

How can I be so sure? Because I've always been a believer in action, and you've already taken action. Here's the first step in the plan:

STEP ONE: DECIDE TO MAKE A CHANGE
You did that when you bought this

book. You are on your way. Take a picture of yourself now, because you'll want to take another picture later, after you've gotten in shape. (And I hope you'll let me include your pictures in a future book or infomercial.) Now take some of those measurements you don't like taking. Don't worry; in a few weeks, you're going to *love* doing this part. For the body measurements, you measure at the fullest point for everything except the waist, which you measure at the thinnest point (but don't suck in). You can use your blood pressure and cholesterol numbers from a recent medical checkup. Check your heart rate while at rest by sitting comfortably in a chair, in view of a clock, putting two fingers to the pulse in your neck, and counting the beats in one minute. If you have diabetes, check your glucose level. Or you can schedule an appointment with your doctor to check these numbers. (Of course, before beginning any exercise program, you should consult your physician about any health concerns you have.) Write your numbers down in the left column. In six weeks, you'll fill in the right column.

Step one is done! Step two is only a teensy-weensy bit harder.

Step Two: Walk Today

That's it. The first thing you do when you open your eyes is ask yourself, When will I walk today? Try walking for fifteen minutes. Couldn't be simpler. I know you can do it. More important, *you* know you can do it. I don't care if you turn on your favorite music or TV show and walk to that, if you head outside and do a trip around the block, or if you pop in my one-mile video and walk with me. It all works! Start off slowly for the first few minutes to let your muscles warm up and to allow your heart rate to rise slowly, increase your pace a bit for the middle of the walk, and then slow down for the last minute or two to cool down.

Pow. Just like that, you've improved your health and your life.

If you haven't yet learned about all the great changes starting to take place in your body because of this walk, this might be a good time to read chapter 3, "The Miracle of Exercise." If you don't want to clutter up your brain right now, just stick to the walking. After all, you get the benefits whether you read about them or not!

If you have any questions about walking posture or technique, turn back to part II, "The Exercises." You'll see how I do it, and I'll give you some tips about how to get the most out of your walk.

For tips on proper clothing and shoes, see chapter 4.

Once you have tried your first walk, you have already completed day one of my six-week program. And that, my friend, means you are ready for the next step.

Step Three: Keep Walking

You'll find the next two weeks of the Walk Diet just as easy because you'll gradually work up to everything. Flip ahead if you like and see what the plan is for

DATE _____   DATE _____
WEIGHT _____   WEIGHT _____

TAPE MEASUREMENTS

UPPER ARM _____ INCHES   UPPER ARM _____ INCHES

CHEST _____ INCHES   CHEST _____ INCHES

WAIST _____ INCHES   WAIST _____ INCHES

HIPS _____ INCHES   HIPS _____ INCHES

THIGH _____ INCHES   THIGH _____ INCHES

HEALTH

BLOOD PRESSURE _____   BLOOD PRESSURE _____

CHOLESTEROL _____   CHOLESTEROL _____

HEART RATE _____   HEART RATE _____

GLUCOSE _____   GLUCOSE _____

BEFORE   AFTER

PLACE YOUR PHOTO HERE   PLACE YOUR PHOTO HERE

each day—it's all laid out for you. In Week 1, we'll concentrate on one-mile walks. You even get Sunday off! I also introduce the first of what I call "Walk Boosters"— simple lifestyle tips that boost the health benefits gained from walking.

At first, don't worry about making any other changes in your life. You've done enough for the moment. Eat as you normally do. Sleep as you normally do. Stress out as you normally do! Your only goal is to establish walking as a part of your routine. You'll probably feel more energy and optimism from day one. After two full weeks of walking, you'll be ready to mix in the next component of your program.

STEP FOUR: STRENGTH TRAINING

I know, strength training sounds scary. Even I get images of ripped guys in the gym and Arnold Schwarzenegger bodybuilding contests. I shiver at the thought of complicated exercises to learn, weird contortions, and dangerous weights over my head. Which is why my version of strength training is completely different. Mine involves nothing more complicated than doing simple arm exercises while you walk. A pair of one-pound weights in your hands and, without even realizing it, you're doing strength training. It's that easy! The benefits of strength training are enormous, from stronger bones and increased metabolism to a firmer, slimmer upper body.

Beginning with Week 3 of the Walk Diet, you'll work some basic strength training into your walks. Because you do it while you walk, this means no additional time commitment on your part. By the end of this third week, the definition in your upper body and the slimming in your lower half will be obvious. Your energy and confidence will be at an all-time high.

STEP FIVE: SELF-ACCEPTANCE

As you enter Week 4 of the Walk Diet, you'll be walking one to three miles per day with ease and using some resistance training to flatten your abs and hips while you walk. You'll feel great and the pounds will be melting away. *Now's* the time for that introspection. I agree with the motivation gurus: Accepting ourselves as we are and escaping our self-destructive modes of behavior really are the keys to permanent change and success. With a few weeks of walking under your belt, your body is now ready to deal with such issues; time for your mind to follow. With your groove back, you can take a look at the factors that forced you into bad habits in the first place and take the necessary steps to change them in order to align your lifestyle with your goals and make them come true. I'll suggest some mental exercises to get you started. Along with that, I'll give you some wonderful ideas for putting the enthusiasm you're feeling into words.

STEP SIX: FINISH STRONG

The last two weeks of the Walk Diet are all about following through. Without pushing yourself too hard, you'll kick your walking into high gear to see just what you're capable of. You'll be amazed as the miles pile up and the waistline goes down. You'll start to wonder who that person was four weeks ago who didn't know if she could walk a single mile. When you catch sight of yourself in mirrors, you'll think, Do I really look that different, or is it all in my head? Here's a secret: The answer to both is yes.

STEP SEVEN: REWARD

Completing the Walk Diet is a time for rejoicing. When you reach this point, you've made an incredible commitment to health and longevity. You've enriched your life and the lives of those who rely on you. Time for a reward. Small rewards are included each week of the program, but this is the time for a biggie. You've earned it. A new wardrobe, a weekend for two in Aruba—don't hold back.

STEP EIGHT: CREATING THE LIFE YOU LOVE

After you complete the Walk Diet, you'll have a new body on your hands, a new attitude, and from this place of strength you can take the opportunity to re-create your life. Walking is now a part of who you are. It would be hard work to break this habit—and you're not about to do that. What else do you need to do to make the most of your time here on Earth? If you haven't already done so, this can be a good time to read part IV of this book, "Making Life Work." It can help you to start addressing the negative stress factors in your life that affect your behavior and happiness, and to realize that life can work the other way around: By loving who you are and asserting yourself in the world, you can be a force of happiness and goodness for others.

And that's it. If you stick to the plan and don't try to rush things, you won't find one bit of it hard. In fact, it's fun—I wouldn't have been doing this for twenty-five years if it wasn't!

Beyond the first six weeks, I'll help you customize your own program to keep you walking and thinking positively for the rest of your life. Do you walk best with a buddy? Do you want to push yourself up to four miles per day? Help others get started? Walk a marathon? It's all there if you want it.

Remember, this all starts from simply walking for fifteen minutes. If you can handle that, you can handle every step in this book. Come on, let me walk you through it.

Walking Wonder

Jill Wilder

FREEPORT, PENNSYLVANIA

Lost 175 pounds

I am a forty-three-year-old vice president of a software company. I have had weight issues and migraine headaches my entire life. I've always wanted to be thinner and feel better, but figured it just wasn't possible for me.

I am thrilled to tell you that I am on my way to being the person I have always wanted to be! I have lost 175 pounds in the past two years following a sensible diet plan and using Leslie's program, and I haven't had a single migraine since I started. I feel great and can do things I never thought possible. The most wonderful thing is that feeling better happened very quickly. Within a couple of weeks I was more active, more flexible, and ready to tackle anything that came my way.

I decided to tackle my weight issues in October 2001. I raise my sister's four children in my home. Being a role model to the children is very important to me, yet here I was unable to make a vital change in my own life. I purchased Leslie's tapes and started to eat sensibly. At first, I could barely make a half mile, but I stuck with it. In a very short period of time I was able to easily make the half mile and started to work on a mile. I have learned to take things at a reasonable pace with small goals. I can't believe how fantastic I feel today! I now walk two or three times a day using Leslie's program and have many friends and coworkers who walk with me. I can't say enough about how much a simple 15 minutes of walking can do for your attitude and outlook on life.

I now have to allow extra time wherever I go just to handle all the compliments and questions from people about how I did it. My kids are so proud of me. But most important, they now realize they can accomplish anything, just the way I did!

8. How to Use the Walk Diet Day Pages

We all learned it in kindergarten: The best way to go through life is using the buddy system. Everything is more fun if you hold someone else's hand. For the six weeks of the Walk Diet, I'm going to be your buddy. By using the Day Pages in the Walk Diet program guide, you'll have me beside you each and every day, motivating you, instructing you, and giving you valuable tips to make getting in shape that much easier. The Day Pages allow you to set your goals for each day, track your progress, and see exactly what lies ahead in the coming weeks. They also help remind you to do the Walk Boosters, which let you boost the health benefits of walking to a whole new level.

If you already walk more than ten miles per week, use the "PowerWalking" chapter to modify the daily workouts to a level that will challenge you. You'll still want to use the Day Pages to track your progress and to learn the valuable tips and techniques for bringing joy and success to all facets of your life.

THE WEEK PAGE

Each week of the Day Pages begins with a Week Page. On this page, I explain the theme we'll be focusing on that week and give you the running total of how many miles you've walked. You'll be amazed how fast that number climbs! I also ask you to jot down what you think your accomplishments were the previous week, and what your goals are for the upcoming one. Don't skip this part! You may feel no need to reflect on your walking, but it makes it all feel much more *real*. And don't limit the accomplishments you list to walking-related ones. Those are important, but so are all your other daily achievements. And they are all connected. If you got a raise at work or went on a date, mention it. You may be surprised at how productive your week was, but you won't even realize it unless you write it all down. Everything in life is connected. You aren't walking to become a better walker; you're walking to get fit. And you're getting fit so that a world of new options opens up to you. So you can hike in a state park. Wear the latest fashion trends. Roughhouse with your kids or grandkids. Life is too complicated to assign cause and effect, but I think you'll find that as you walk more, your weekly accomplishments fill up and spill off the page. So please *do* this part. It may become your favorite task of all!

Please also write in your goals for the week. Again, don't limit this to your walking goals. Psychologists know that if we write down our intentions, we are much more likely to follow through with them. The physical act of committing them to paper helps change the intentions from fuzzy ideas to specific goals. Then we can't forget that we intended to do them in the first place.

For those who prefer to walk with my videos, I list suggestions on each Week Page for ones that match the walking and strength-training goals for that week. But please remember that you are always free to mix and match, to substitute other strength-training equipment for what I recommend for a particular day, or to go with your favorite video instead. Ultimately, you know best what you need and how hard you should push yourself.

THE WALK BOOSTER

After the Week Page comes your Walk Booster for the week. These are special lifestyle tips that supercharge the health benefits you get from walking. They are all simple tasks, such as taking a multivitamin or drinking more water, but the changes they can make in your health and energy are profound.

THE DAY PAGES

The heart of the Walk Diet is found in the Day Pages. Each day of the week, each week of the program, I give you a little pep talk, along with your walking assignment for that day. Beginning with Week 3, I mix in a strength-training component, as well. You have many options for tracking how far you walk. I provide mileage, a time goal, and a steps goal, so you can pick what works for you.

I can't overemphasize the importance of the next line on the Day Pages. It may look small, may seem like no big deal, but let me tell you, it is your key to success. I'm talking about the line where it says, "When will I walk today?" Remember how I explained why it is important to write your goals down, even if it feels a bit silly? The same goes for this simple goal. First thing in the morning (or even better, the night *before*), I want you to open up your Day Pages to that day, commit to a time to walk, and write it in the book. We all know how our days get filled up; you are much more likely to walk if you plan ahead for a specific time and write it down. This moves your intentions out of la-la land and into the real world. I actually like to sit down on Sunday night and plan my walks for the entire week. That way, I already have the time blocked out in case unexpected meetings and invitations come up.

When you do walk, please check off the "Did I walk today?" line on your Day Page. Call me crazy, but I love making a "To Do" list and then checking items off one by one as I plow through them. Here's your chance to do the same. You get a little hit of endorphins with every check. In addition to the walking, you can keep track of your multivitamin and water consumption. As you near the end of the six weeks, you can flip back and see how you've improved.

The Tip of the day features small strategies and lifestyle changes that my friends, coworkers, and I have found invaluable for helping us stick to our routines and stay sane in general. Take it from personal experience—they really work!

I've saved some room on each Day Page for you to record how you felt after your walk. If it was a breeze and you were so revved up that you kept going and cleaned out the garage, write that down. If you were pooped halfway through and had to stop, write that down, too. If you have ideas for a slightly different approach you could take tomorrow, jot them down. It all helps to compile a record of your progress and generate insights about how to improve. If you happen to get blood pressure or cholesterol readings during this time (or glucose levels for diabetics), you can track those here, too.

The last thing on the Day Pages is the one you might roll your eyes at. I give you a line to record "A Beautiful Thing" you noticed that day. This can be anything that strikes you. It could be a perfect yellow rose. It could be a cat curled blissfully in a sunny window, or a little boy and his grandmother playing in the park. No, I haven't gone soft and, no, I'm not the type of person who turns the dots on all her *i*'s into hearts. Every day is a glass that can be half-full or half-empty, depending on how you look at it. Weighed down by the stresses of daily life, it becomes too easy for us to start seeing only the empty side. Actively looking for beauty in each day is simply a way of training your mind to see the full side of life. But it doesn't work to make a broad statement, such as, "Today, I'm going to look on the bright side." The mind doesn't work that way. Just as you become physically fit slowly, by taking one step after another, you become emotionally fit by making small changes that will eventually transform the way you see yourself and the world. Start slowly. Feel free to say, "This is so silly" if you want, as long as you do it. By Week 6, you may find yourself noticing more beautiful things each day than you can possibly record. And that's when you know you've really changed.

So don't laugh. Try it. Finding beauty just may become a lifelong habit.

Sunday Day Pages are different from the rest. Sundays are your free days. You get more benefits from exercise when you give your body regular breaks to recover, and that is what Sundays are for. Do what you want, drink what you want, and don't keep track of anything. You even get a reward! Burnout is less likely this way. Instead of a scheduled routine, on Sundays I give you a general idea for working on your spiritual fitness. Whether this means going to a cathedral or a spa, the goal is to make yourself feel sacred. And if you don't believe *that* is a vital part of your success, then you haven't felt sacred in way too long. Let's get started on changing that.

A Little Learning

After the Day Pages, each week of the Walk Diet concludes with "A Little Learning," minichapters that give you the lowdown on why you are doing what you're doing. Want to understand why exercise makes the body healthier? This is the place to look. Want to know why food diets usually don't work? You'll find out here. These sections aren't long, so anytime during the week when you have a few spare minutes, you can pick up the book, flip to A Little Learning for that week, and come away with a deeper understanding of your body and its mental, physical, and spiritual health.

These sections are not required reading. If you are one of those people who likes to follow a simple program and just cares *that* it works, not why it works, then feel free to skip them. But if you are like me, you'll enjoy seeing the big picture and being able to tell others about why what you're doing makes so much sense.

Oh, and One More Thing . . .

And now is the point in the program where I tell you to pitch any part of the program that isn't working for you. If *anything* in the program is keeping you from walking—drinking the water, focusing on self-affirmation, waiting for a cardinal to visit your feeder so you can record your beautiful thing—then forget about it. The walking is the key. And if the amount of *walking* is stopping you from walking, then cut it in half. Even a little walking makes you healthier than none. While I hope you'll be able to follow along with the amounts recommended in the program and reach a real health milestone, the important thing is for you to be comfortable with the amount of effort, to look forward to it, and to increase your workouts gradually, setting your own pace.

How Long Do I Walk?

Indoor walking has many advantages, but tracking your walks isn't one of them. Walking outdoors usually makes it pretty easy to tell how far you've gone. If you are walking around the block, you can drive the route in your car and get the mileage. And many city parks have walking trails with the mileage listed. If you walk inside, things are slightly more complicated, but we've come up with several foolproof systems! They are explained below. All the walking assignments in the book list times, distances, and steps, so you can use whichever system appeals to you the most.

Timed Walking

Timing yourself with a clock while you walk is about as simple as it gets. Many indoor walkers don't even use a clock because they like to watch TV or listen to music while they walk. They choose a half-hour TV show and walk all the way through it. Or they set their CD player for twenty minutes of music and walk through that. The only decision comes in setting your pace. (Music can be a great pacesetter!) You can walk a very slow one-mile, half-hour walk, or race through two miles of brisk walking in the same time period. To get a sense of how fast you're walking, use this yardstick:

Most fit people walk down a street at about three miles per hour, meaning they do a mile every twenty minutes. Those fast walkers who bustle by you on the sidewalk are going about four miles per hour: a mile every fifteen minutes. It's difficult to walk faster than that without pumping your arms and looking like a racer. If you find that most people pass you when you're walking down a street, you probably walk about two miles per hour: a mile every thirty minutes. That's the minimum speed you should maintain for your indoor walks. Here's a guide to keep in mind:

Leisurely walk:	1 mile in 30 minutes
Moderate walk:	1 mile in 20 minutes
Brisk walk:	1 mile in 15 minutes

I use these terms for the time recommendations on the Day Pages to describe how quickly you should walk. They are only a guideline, however, and you should determine whatever pace feels right to you.

Pedometers

I'm a big fan of pedometers because they take all the guesswork out of walking. Whether you are short or tall, whether you walk fast or slow, a pedometer will tell you exactly how many steps you've taken. It will even convert these steps into miles for you, but why bother? You can just keep all your goals in steps, which are even more accurate. The other great advantage of pedometers is that you can wear them all day to track how many steps you are taking while doing daily activities as well as structured walks. Most of us take about 3,000 steps a day just going about our typical tasks. I recommend 6,000 steps per day (including exercise) as the *minimum* number to maintain health, and 8,000–10,000 per day to achieve weight loss. Walking a mile takes about 2,000 steps. Taking a three-mile walk each day nets you

6,000 steps; add in the 3,000 you get doing everything else and you are up to 9,000: an excellent number for weight loss. Start to do things like using stairs instead of elevators, or walking through malls while shopping, and you'll hit that 10,000 mark, where the pounds disappear faster than you can keep track. Throughout the Walk Diet in this book, I'll give you step goals to strive for. (Just remember that those goals include only your structured walking; you should be doing an additional 3,000 each day just living!)

Video Walking

One of the things so many people like about my videos is that I keep track of time and distance for you. You just match my pace and watch the mile meter at the bottom of the screen as you hit each half-mile mark. You can also follow my moves closely. For those who like this approach, I provide video suggestions for each week of the Walk Diet.

Walking Wonder

Belinda Zamudio

HAMMOND, INDIANA

Lost 47 pounds

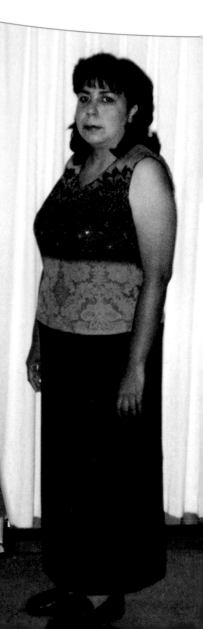

Walk Away the Pounds has changed my life! I started gaining weight shortly after I got married in 1982. I kept getting bigger year by year, until I reached my highest weight, 231 pounds. I was out of control and knew that I needed to do something before it got too late. I tried dieting, but I always gave up when I didn't see immediate results.

In February 2002, I joined Weight Watchers. The group instructor encouraged us to start exercising and mentioned Leslie's program. I hadn't exercised since high school and was scared of trying, but from the way the instructor was describing the program, it sounded like maybe this was something I could do.

I bought my first Walk Away the Pounds tape right after the meeting. The first few times I tried were difficult. I lasted only ten minutes and couldn't even get through the middle of the workout. But I didn't give up. Leslie keeps encouraging you. It almost seems as if she is talking right to you. When I felt I couldn't go on exercising, she would say, "You can do it!" or "C'mon, legs, just a little bit more!" She gave me the strength to go on. I kept at it, and pretty soon I was completing fifteen minutes, then twenty minutes, and then two months later I did the whole tape. I started noticing that I had a lot more energy and my clothes were looser. I'm so excited and look forward to working out every day.

What I like about Leslie's program is that you can do it in the privacy of your home. I was too embarrassed to go to the gym because of my size. I would not be where I am right now without God having given me the strength and Leslie's encouraging words. I have lost a total of forty-seven pounds! I know if I got this far, I can reach my goal of 140 pounds.

9. Week 1

LET'S GET STARTED!

*H*ere *we go!* There is nothing more exciting than the beginning of a wonderful journey, and this promises to be a great one. You need to do only *one* thing this week, and that is walk. Don't think about what you eat, don't think about what you drink, and definitely don't make any other changes in your life. If you overwhelm yourself with too many new goals at once, you won't be able to deal with any of them. Keep it simple this week. Just walk. If you have any questions about form, review the basic moves in chapter 5.

To keep things really simple, your Walk Booster for the week requires no real effort on your part, but it still can make a difference in your health. I want you to take a multivitamin every day. Every supermarket and pharmacy offers plenty to choose from, so just pick one and pop it in with your breakfast juice. You may be surprised how good it makes you feel!

A Little Learning this week explains how just walking for a few minutes a day can trigger changes that help you break free from your old life altogether. You see, there really is a method to my madness, so when you have a few minutes this week, flip to the end of this chapter to find out what it is.

Happy walking, everyone!

TOTAL MILES WALKED: 0	WALK BOOSTER: Multivitamin
NEW MILES THIS WEEK: 6	USEFUL VIDEOS: *Walk With Me*
A LITTLE LEARNING: Breakthrough!	*Heart-Healthy Walk*

TAKING STOCK
My goals for this week are: _____

_____

_____

_____

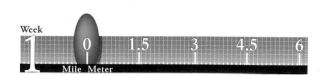

MULTIVITAMIN

Does a daily multivitamin improve your health? You will get as many answers to this question as you can find books, talk-radio shows, and infomercials on the subject. "Pound megadoses of vitamin pills for good health!" says one source. "Don't let anything other than organic, raw foods pass your lips!" says another. I believe the truth lies somewhere in the middle.

If you eat the Little Miss Perfect Diet, with mountains of tomatoes and forests of broccoli at every sitting, you will probably get 100 percent of your recommended daily allowance (RDA) for all vitamins and minerals and won't really need a multivitamin. But who among us eats like that? Yeah, no one I know, either. The rest of us, eating like normal human beings, risk certain vitamin deficiencies. Among many other tasks, vitamins are responsible for regulating the metabolism and the immune system, preventing the breakdown of tissue that can lead to cancer and heart disease, and keeping your nerves and brain functioning properly.

Even if you are eating enough vitamin-rich foods to meet the RDA standards, you might want to take a multivitamin. Those standards were designed to keep people from malnutrition diseases such as scurvy, but they don't take into account vitamins' ability to prevent cancer, cardiovascular disease, and other conditions if taken at higher doses. (Never take *more* than a single multivitamin provides, however. Excessive doses of certain vitamins can *cause* diseases.)

Some vitamin companies may claim that vitamins will give you extra energy, which isn't really true. Vitamins don't produce energy on their own—all your energy comes from the food you eat—but vitamins are essential for your body to convert food into energy and use it, so vitamin deficiencies can result in low energy. If you find your energy level improving after you start taking a multivitamin, it probably means that your body is using the energy from your food more efficiently.

Vitamin supplements may also give us the upper hand in staving off disease, especially as we age. Heart health, immune support, and bone strength benefit the most from supplements, and the vitamins you want to look for are B_6, B_{12}, C, and folic acid. My favorite multivitamins are the Cooper Completes made by Kenneth Cooper (www.coopercomplete.com) and those made by Andrew Weil (www.drweil.com). Cooper's Web site includes an excellent multivitamin for kids. Weil's Vitamin Advisor asks you some basic questions; then he formulates customized pills to suit your needs. Pop your vitamin each morning, and if it makes a difference in your health and energy, keep doing it.

I *told* you this was going to be easy!

WEEK 1   MONDAY

For our very first day, we're simply going to walk one mile. If you've never walked before, this may sound daunting, but you'll find it isn't that far. It will probably take you only thirty minutes or so, but don't worry how long it takes; just aim to complete the whole mile. We tend to think of anything measured in miles as "car distance"—"The beach? Oh, it's a mile away."—but that will all change with this program. By the end, you'll be saying things like "That movie theater is only three miles away. Let's walk." And it all starts today with that first mile.

WALK:	1 mile
	30 leisurely minutes
	2,000 steps
STRENGTH:	Nothing this week

WHEN WILL I WALK TODAY? _____

DID I WALK TODAY? ☐

DID I TAKE MY MULTIVITAMIN? ☐

Tip Never forget the warm-up and cool-down parts of your walk. Warming up gets fluid into your joints and muscles, so you are limber and can avoid injury. Warm muscles can hold more oxygen than cold muscles, so you don't run out of breath as fast. Cooling down at the end of a walk allows your body to filter waste products created by exercise so your muscles won't be sore the next day.

HOW DID I FEEL?

_____

_____

_____

_____

A BEAUTIFUL THING

_____

_____

_____

_____

WEEK 1   TUESDAY

Congratulations! You did your first mile! And you know what? That will be the hardest mile you ever do. To prove it, walk the same mile at the same pace today and see how much easier it feels.

WALK:	1 mile
	30 leisurely minutes
	2,000 steps
STRENGTH:	Nothing this week

WHEN WILL I WALK TODAY? _____

DID I WALK TODAY? ☐

DID I TAKE MY MULTIVITAMIN? ☐

Tip What you wear on your feet makes a big difference in comfort during and after a walk. Quality sneakers and socks will keep your feet drier, well supported, and pain-free. (A lot of misinformation about shoes and socks exists, so please read my section on gear in chapter 4 for the real scoop.)

HOW DID I FEEL?

_____

_____

_____

_____

A BEAUTIFUL THING

_____

_____

_____

_____

WEEK 1   WEDNESDAY

Amazing how much easier that walk was yesterday. Your body is already responding. Do one more mile today and focus on pace. Try to complete the walk in twenty-five minutes. Don't worry if you take longer. Your endurance and strength will build over time.

WALK:	1 mile
	25 leisurely minutes
	2,000 steps
STRENGTH:	Nothing this week

WHEN WILL I WALK TODAY? _____

DID I WALK TODAY? ☐

DID I TAKE MY MULTIVITAMIN? ☐

Tip Lower your standards! Never let housework be your reason for not walking. If it is, your priorities are backward. I have walked past more smelly socks, sinks of dishes, and dusty cupboards than I can count. If I hadn't, I wouldn't be here today. I'd still be at home scrubbing!

HOW DID I FEEL?

_____

_____

_____

_____

A BEAUTIFUL THING

_____

_____

_____

_____

WEEK 1   THURSDAY

One day in the middle of each week, you get to recharge your batteries. This gives you a change of pace and keeps your routine from seeming stale. That way, you stay motivated. Today is your first of these unstructured days. I call them "unstructured" because, while you don't do any "official" walks, you are supposed to stay active so that the calorie burning continues. Anytime you have the chance to do something physical today, seize it. Crank through the laundry. Play soccer with your kid. Do some gardening. It all adds up! If you have a pedometer, wear it from the time you get out of bed until you go to sleep and see how many steps you get in. People typically walk 3,000 steps in the course of a day without exercise, so with an extra mile of unstructured walking, you should aim for 5,000.

WALK:	Unstructured
	5,000 steps all day
STRENGTH:	Nothing this week

WHEN WILL I WALK TODAY? _____

DID I WALK TODAY? ☐

DID I TAKE MY MULTIVITAMIN? ☐

Tip I recommend pedometers, or step counters, as the best way of telling exactly how much exercise you get during a day. See my section on gear in chapter 4 for information about buying one.

How did I feel?

_____

_____

_____

_____

A beautiful thing

_____

_____

_____

_____

WEEK 1   FRIDAY

Love those one-mile walks! Try to complete your mile in twenty minutes. If it takes twenty-five, that's still good. The important thing is to keep improving. Picking up the pace, even a little, burns a lot of extra calories. But don't kill yourself—save something for your first two-miler tomorrow!

WALK:	1 mile
	20 moderate minutes
	2,000 steps
STRENGTH:	Nothing this week

WHEN WILL I WALK TODAY? _____

DID I WALK TODAY? ☐

DID I TAKE MY MULTIVITAMIN? ☐

Tip Try walking first thing in the morning. For lots of us, that's the only time of day we aren't behind schedule! Morning walks kick your energy and metabolism into high gear right away, so you burn extra calories all day long.

How did I feel?

_____

_____

_____

_____

A beautiful thing

_____

_____

_____

_____

WEEK 1 SATURDAY

Those one-mile walks are going down pretty smoothly, huh? Think you can do two today? If not, that's fine. Do what you can do. Exercise should always be fun and refreshing. If it's exhausting or something you dread, you're pushing too hard. Cut back. The health and weight-loss benefits come from moderate exercise, not from punishing ourselves. But I think you are ready for two miles. When you hit that one-mile mark, see how you feel. Still going strong? Then that second mile will go even faster than the first. On the other hand, you may find that you slow down a lot for the second mile, so I've built some extra time in for that one.

> **WALK:**   2 miles
>   50 leisurely minutes
>   4,000 steps
> **STRENGTH:** Nothing this week

WHEN WILL I WALK TODAY? _____

DID I WALK TODAY? ☐

DID I TAKE MY MULTIVITAMIN? ☐

Tip Walking with headphones is one of the classic ways to make workout time fly. Listen to your favorite tunes or try one of my audiotapes (see Resources).

HOW DID I FEEL?

_____

_____

_____

_____

A BEAUTIFUL THING

_____

_____

_____

_____

WEEK 1   SUNDAY

Whew! You did it! I *knew* you could. Was that two-mile walk hard yesterday, or did you sail through it? Either way, you put a week of walking under your belt and you are a changed person already. Now it's time to *recharge*. Sundays are our day for resting from walking. Stop and smell the roses, take a break from physical fitness, and instead work on *spiritual fitness* by praying, going to church, spending time with family, cooking beautiful meals, or whatever it is that fills your heart with gladness.

Don't keep track of any of your Walk Boosters on Sunday, either. Anything that you do for too long without a break can start to feel like a chore, so if you want to take your multivitamin, to keep your eyes peeled for that beautiful moment, or to do any of the other suggestions, go ahead, but don't feel compelled to, and don't worry about writing anything down. It's your day! Enjoy!

As part of that enjoyment, a reward is in order. Treat yourself to something that will help you complete the program. A subscription to one of those great walking magazines, perhaps? New sneakers? A DVD player? If it helps you stay motivated, it's worth it.

BREAKTHROUGH!

We all know when we're in a rut. Unfortunately, this doesn't make it any easier to break out! The classic characteristics of a rut are patterns of negative thinking and behavior that reinforce each other and make us dig ourselves in deeper and deeper. We stop exercising, we get out of shape, and this makes it harder to start again. Lack of exercise leads to weight gain and depression. Feeling this weight upon us—literally and mentally—we are less likely than ever to start exercising again. This is followed by more weight gain, and the cycle feeds on itself over and over.

We've all been stuck in similar patterns. When the rut gets too deep, we eventually turn somewhere for help. But whether it is to fitness, weight-loss, or self-help, we are usually told to embrace an impossible approach. The self-help books tell us to change ourselves through self-reflection and "soul-work." Even leading weight-loss books often tell us to accept ourselves as we are before beginning on a program. This sounds sensible, but people in the depths of a funk find it almost impossible to do this through force of mind alone. The negative mental patterns are just too strong.

Other weight-loss programs skip the soul-searching and cut straight to the workout. They ask you to embrace some complicated, intimidating, or overly strenuous exercise program. Sure, if followed, this program will lead to weight loss and improved self-image. But when the chips are down, few people are ready to tackle an extensive program.

These approaches are just too much, too soon. If you picture the rut you are in as a river canyon, they are saying, "There is a way out, and it is really close. Just free-climb this thousand-foot cliff next to you!"

Well, thanks, but if I could do that, I'd already be on Everest by now!

So what to do? If you could just clear away these mental cobwebs, you'd probably have the energy to start exercising. And if you were exercising every day, the cobwebs might blow away on their own. But how to begin?

The secret lies in breaking the negative patterns that bind you. These patterns can seem as strong as a straitjacket, impossible to break through force of will, but if you know how, like Houdini, you can slip out without fighting at all.

Our minds and bodies are woven together in an incredibly close relationship. Anything that affects one affects the other. Few people realize it, but to change negative thinking patterns, it is often easier simply to change your *physical* patterns. Study after study have shown that certain types of physical behavior can take you to a totally different mental state. Your senses start feeding different information to your brain, your breathing and blood flow are different, and suddenly you're in a different place.

It's like jump-starting a car. Usually the brain, like a car battery, is responsible for triggering the initial impulse that gets the body started. But at those times when the brain is out of juice, if you can get the body moving, the energy flows the other way and charges up the brain. Then all sorts of good things happen. New ideas pop. Creativity flows. A sense of well-being suffuses you. And things that seemed hard or impossible start to seem downright easy.

Psychologists call this state of mind "flow," or "peak experience," and we've all experienced it at times. We lose ourselves so completely in what we're doing that our mind gets free to go a-wandering on its own. And that's when a lot of good insights about ourselves come into focus.

There are many ways to access this state, but the very easiest is through repetitive exercise. Usually fifteen minutes is enough. You don't even need to leave your living room. Just a week of walking and you will have broken your old patterns. Will you lose significant weight in a week? No. You may lose a little, but, more important, you'll have a whole new platform of confidence and emotional stability, from which you can look down on the terrain of your life and act. You'll see the rut you've been stuck in stretching away behind you, and you'll see a new way out of it. Not the steep cliff rising above you, but a *gradual path* you never knew existed, one that meanders slowly up the other side of the cliff to the plateau. From there, you can see all the possible paths, all your choices. You can see which fall into new ruts, and which don't, and you can make your choice about where you want to go in life from this enlightened place.

C'mon, Leslie, you're thinking, that's a pretty big claim to make for just putting one foot in front of the other. And you're right. I'm not claiming that walking on its own will change your life. *You* are going to change your life. Walking is just the easiest vehicle for doing so.

There is even science to back up this idea. Researchers have found that simple repetitive exercises such as walking trigger a release of nitric oxide throughout the body. This chemical dilates blood vessels, reducing blood pressure and allowing more blood and nutrients to be pumped to the cells. Its greatest effect may be in the brain. By permitting the free flow of neurotransmitters in the brain, nitric oxide alters brain chemistry, improving memory, mood, and performance. It literally creates a new you! And this whole process happens while you walk. You probably aren't even aware of it—though with experience, you'll recognize the feelings as your brain starts to perk up and think creatively halfway through your walk.

Toward the end of this first week of walking, try to pay some attention to your mental state. Are you feeling more energetic? Is your problem-solving ability at work on the rise? Are you looking forward to walking next week?

My bet is that you are. Which means you have broken your old patterns once and for all.

Walking Wonder

Linda Anthony
WEST NEWTON, PENNSYLVANIA

Lost 120 pounds

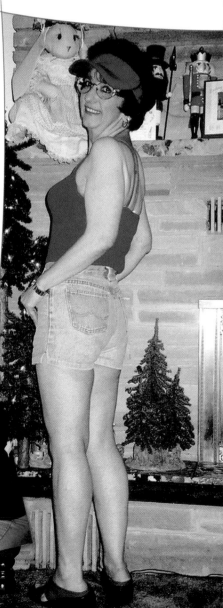

In January 2002, I was diagnosed with diabetes. I weighed 240 pounds, my sugar level was over 200, and I was scared to death. My mother had gone blind and eventually died from diabetes, and I feared that I was next. With that in mind, I participated in a weight-loss study at the University of Pittsburgh Medical Center. The nutritionists there are huge believers in exercise and they recommended Leslie's program. So when Leslie made an appearance at my local mall, I went to check her out. I was so motivated, I got up onstage and participated! From that day, I was hooked.

Who would have thought I could exercise in my tiny living room, let alone enjoy it? But I did, immensely! I quickly worked up to three miles and really missed it if I didn't get to walk during the day. My stress level went down, both at work and at home, and my menopause mood swings leveled off. One thing I didn't expect was that my concentration improved. I feel terrific *and have so much energy!*

Today, I weigh 120 pounds. My sugar level is 90–100: a normal reading! I take no *diabetic medication—walking and diet control my diabetes completely. My lifestyle has improved, as well. Believe it or not, I've been in three fashion shows, where the emcee announced my weight loss. I'm even president of the West Newton VFD Auxiliary. I'd never have had the confidence to pursue these things in the past. This exercise program literally saved my life.*

10. Week 2

WATER, WATER EVERYWHERE

Hey, six miles logged already. You are off to a great start. Now this week, we will walk, walk, walk. You should start to notice a real difference. Energy up? Falling asleep faster? It's all from that walking. Remind yourself of this as you push through a few extra miles this week.

Now we are going to take your health to a whole new level. Remember when I told you that you wouldn't have to think about what you eat on this "diet"? Well, that's true, but what you *drink* is another story. You can still drink soda or coffee, but your Walk Booster for this week is going to be eight glasses a day of pure, delicious water. Why? you ask. Read on. A Little Learning will tell you everything you need to know about why water is in many ways the number-one key to good health.

TOTAL MILES WALKED: 6	**WALK BOOSTER:** Water
NEW MILES THIS WEEK: 9	**USEFUL VIDEOS:** *Walk With Me*
A LITTLE LEARNING: Water Is Life	*Heart-Healthy Walk*
	Super Fat Burning

TAKING STOCK

My accomplishments last week were: ⸺⸺⸺⸺⸺⸺⸺

⸺⸺⸺⸺⸺⸺⸺⸺⸺⸺⸺⸺⸺⸺⸺

⸺⸺⸺⸺⸺⸺⸺⸺⸺⸺⸺⸺⸺⸺⸺

⸺⸺⸺⸺⸺⸺⸺⸺⸺⸺⸺⸺⸺⸺⸺

My goals for this week are: ⸺⸺⸺⸺⸺⸺⸺⸺

⸺⸺⸺⸺⸺⸺⸺⸺⸺⸺⸺⸺⸺⸺⸺

⸺⸺⸺⸺⸺⸺⸺⸺⸺⸺⸺⸺⸺⸺⸺

⸺⸺⸺⸺⸺⸺⸺⸺⸺⸺⸺⸺⸺⸺⸺

⸺⸺⸺⸺⸺⸺⸺⸺⸺⸺⸺⸺⸺⸺⸺

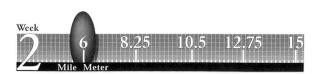

Week 2 | 6 8.25 10.5 12.75 15 | Mile Meter

WATER

You can't get something for nothing, but this week you're going to come pretty darn close. Your Walk Booster for Week 2 requires no time commitment or change in routine on your part. You don't even have to buy anything. Just make sure you drink eight glasses a day of good clean water. Then watch the health benefits pile up. If this water ends up replacing high-calorie drinks—sodas, juices, or coffee with sugar—then you will lose a lot of extra weight. But I'm not even going to ask you to do that, because the main reason I want you to drink water is for health reasons, not weight loss. Feel free to drink the eight glasses of water in addition to everything else you drink. (Of course, you may start to slosh when you walk.) But this can be another great example of a good new habit forcing out a bad old habit: Chances are that if you drink your water first thing in the morning and *before* you get thirsty, you will end up drinking much less of the bad stuff.

Eight glasses a day is a lot to keep track of. Starting this week, I provide a checklist for each day's water. That way, you'll know if you hit dinnertime and still have four glasses to guzzle. Try to space it out. A Little Learning will give you tips for doing just that, in addition to telling you all the amazing things water does for your body.

By now, you may be starting to get the sense that these Walk Boosters are going to be *really* easy. And they are. That's the point! If you think fitness is all about hardship and self-sacrifice—"no pain, no gain"—then you've been bamboozled by the diet industry. They want you to think that big effort (heavy-duty workouts, hard-core diets, or pills) is necessary for big change. The message that I want to spread far and wide is that a few little changes can have *big* effects. And one of the biggest will begin this week as you surf to good health on a wave of water.

WEEK 2 MONDAY

Last Monday started with one mile, so today let's do two. Your body is primed after that day off; plus, it desperately wants to walk off that death-by-chocolate cake your in-laws brought over for Sunday supper. Gotta love 'em; they meant well. The beauty of it is that you don't need to feel guilty for that cake; just do some extra miles this week and it'll be ancient history! Now do you see why an exercise diet beats a food diet hands down?

WALK: 2 miles
45 leisurely minutes
4,000 steps
STRENGTH: Nothing this week

WHEN WILL I WALK TODAY? _____

DID I WALK TODAY? ☐

DID I TAKE MY MULTIVITAMIN? ☐

DID I DRINK MY WATER? ☐

WATER LOG:

WAKE-UP   BREAKFAST   PREWALK   POSTWALK   LUNCH   ANYTIME   DINNER   ANYTIME

Tip To sculpt all the muscles in your core—thighs, buns, back, and abs—make sure you do my whole range of walking moves. Read through the step-by-step exercises in part II to incorporate them into your workout routine.

HOW DID I FEEL?

_____

_____

_____

_____

A BEAUTIFUL THING

_____

_____

_____

_____

Walk Log   **Date** _____

WEEK 2   TUESDAY

Did you get your eight glasses in yesterday? Don't worry about it; as long as you were close, that's a good start. And remember: practice makes perfect, so aim for all eight today and just do one mile—but try to make it an eighteen-minute mile. You can do it!

WALK: 1 mile
            18 moderate minutes
            2,000 steps
STRENGTH: Nothing this week

WHEN WILL I WALK TODAY? _____

DID I WALK TODAY? ☐

DID I TAKE MY MULTIVITAMIN? ☐

DID I DRINK MY WATER? ☐

WATER LOG:
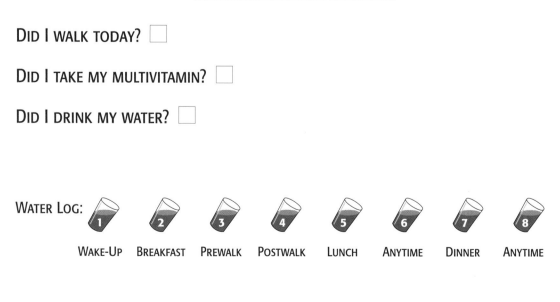

| WAKE-UP | BREAKFAST | PREWALK | POSTWALK | LUNCH | ANYTIME | DINNER | ANYTIME |
| 1 | 2 | 3 | 4 | 5 | 6 | 7 | 8 |

Tip If the best time for you to walk is on your lunch break, you can use my one-mile Walk at Work DVD right on your computer. The U.S. Department of Health and Human Services liked this idea so much, they ordered one thousand copies for their entire staff!

HOW DID I FEEL?

_____

_____

_____

_____

A BEAUTIFUL THING

_____

_____

_____

_____

WEEK 2   WEDNESDAY

Today is a good day for a break from structured walking, because the rest of the week is going to intensify. Look for little walking opportunities throughout your day. You'll be amazed at how many extra steps a day you take once you look for ways to extend your walking instead of avoiding it.

WALK:	Unstructured 6,000 steps all day
STRENGTH:	Nothing this week

WHEN WILL I WALK TODAY? _____

DID I WALK TODAY? ☐

DID I TAKE MY MULTIVITAMIN? ☐

DID I DRINK MY WATER? ☐

WATER LOG:

1	2	3	4	5	6	7	8
WAKE-UP	BREAKFAST	PREWALK	POSTWALK	LUNCH	ANYTIME	DINNER	ANYTIME

Tip Take a trip to the mall, park at one end, and make sure you visit the store at the far end. That round-trip alone is worth a couple of miles of walking! Having any sort of shop in mind as your destination for an outdoor walk is a great way to stay motivated.

How did I feel?

_____

_____

_____

_____

A beautiful thing

_____

_____

_____

_____

Date _____

WEEK 2   THURSDAY

Did you hit your eighteen-minute mile on Tuesday? Think you can do it twice today? Aim to finish in thirty-six minutes. (By the way, how's the house? Messy? Good for you!)

WALK: 2 miles
         36 moderate minutes
         4,000 steps
STRENGTH: Nothing this week

WHEN WILL I WALK TODAY? _____

DID I WALK TODAY? ☐

DID I TAKE MY MULTIVITAMIN? ☐

DID I DRINK MY WATER? ☐

WATER LOG: 1 2 3 4 5 6 7 8

WAKE-UP   BREAKFAST   PREWALK   POSTWALK   LUNCH   ANYTIME   DINNER   ANYTIME

Tip One of the most important parts of this program happens when you *miss* a walk. Don't tell me it won't happen. As you carry walking with you into your new life, eventually a day will come when suddenly it's ten o'clock at night and you haven't walked! When that happens, I want you to get out your time machine immediately, teleport yourself back to the beginning of the day, and walk.

What's that? You don't have a time machine? Then *don't worry about the walk*. Move on. Don't stress over things in the past, and don't try to double your walks tomorrow, or you'll exhaust yourself. Just keep going. Perfect attendance is not our goal.

If you find motivation becoming an ongoing problem, slide your eyes over to chapter 23, "The Motivation Station," and get a fill-up on techniques to keep you going.

HOW DID I FEEL?

_____

_____

_____

_____

A BEAUTIFUL THING

_____

_____

_____

_____

WEEK 2   FRIDAY

How is your energy level? That combination of good hydration and steady exercise should keep you humming along on an even keel throughout the day. No slumps caused by dehydration or flagging metabolism. Today you're going to breeze through a plain-old one-miler for the final time. Marvel at how that felt like work just ten days ago. And an easy day allows you to rest up for your next challenge: your first three-miler tomorrow!

WALK:	1 mile
	18 moderate minutes
	2,000 steps
STRENGTH:	Nothing this week

WHEN WILL I WALK TODAY? _____

DID I WALK TODAY? ☐

DID I TAKE MY MULTIVITAMIN? ☐

DID I DRINK MY WATER? ☐

WATER LOG:

1	2	3	4	5	6	7	8
WAKE-UP	BREAKFAST	PREWALK	POSTWALK	LUNCH	ANYTIME	DINNER	ANYTIME

Tip If you sometimes walk at work on your lunch break, don't lug the same pair of sneakers back and forth with you each day. You're bound to forget them sometimes. Buy a second pair for the office—it's the cheapest investment in your health you can make!

How did I feel?

_____

_____

_____

_____

A beautiful thing

_____

_____

_____

_____

WEEK 2   SATURDAY

Here is a chance to feel incredibly proud of yourself. Today, you will walk three miles for the first time—as far as you ever go during the Walk Diet. Once you master today, the rest is downhill. Don't worry about pace; try to finish the three miles in whatever time you need. If you are following my videos and can't keep up, don't worry about it. Slow down to what feels right to you and know that you'll soon be keeping up with ease.

WALK: 3 miles
         60 moderate minutes
         6,000 steps
STRENGTH: Nothing this week

WHEN WILL I WALK TODAY? _____

DID I WALK TODAY? ☐

DID I TAKE MY MULTIVITAMIN? ☐

DID I DRINK MY WATER? ☐

WATER LOG:

WAKE-UP   BREAKFAST   PREWALK   POSTWALK   LUNCH   ANYTIME   DINNER   ANYTIME

Tip Don't be one of those people who say, "I've got no time to exercise" but then spend five hours a week sitting in the bleachers watching their kids' soccer games. That's five potential hours of walking. Save your aching buns and spend that time walking up and down the sideline, following the action. (Just don't yell at the ref!)

HOW DID I FEEL?

_____

_____

_____

_____

A BEAUTIFUL THING

_____

_____

_____

_____

WEEK 2   SUNDAY

Two weeks and counting! Time for another free day. Relax. Do something for someone else to charge up those spiritual batteries. That's the best reward of all. Volunteer at a nursing home or a day-care center. Drop in on a friend just to make her feel good. Put a gift in the mail to a cousin or a nephew or niece. So much of who we are in life comes from our web of connections to other people, yet this web is easy to ignore because it doesn't press on us like work, house chores, or even the latest episode of our favorite show. But those connections reward us in a way the other things don't. Reach out, and you'll feel the hands of community reaching back to you in a hundred guises.

WATER IS LIFE

So many people who decide to take charge of their health begin to exercise, and even eat more consciously, but they forget about water. This is putting the cart before the horse, because water is the foundation of life and health. One simple fact can illustrate this: Your body can go months without solid food, but more than a couple of days without water and you are in deep trouble.

No wonder. Women's bodies are 60 percent water, and water regulates every process in our bodies, from digestion and blood circulation to sweating, energy supply, and elimination of toxins. Water is life—for every cell.

If I could prescribe exercise for every overweight, unhealthy, or depressed person in America, the hospitals would be half-empty. If I could get all Americans to drink eight glasses of water a day, you could shut down some of those hospitals for good.

Eight glasses is what doctors recommend we get each day, but few of us do. We are all so busy with work, house chores, the kids' fast-paced schedules, and the endless other unexpected tasks that spring up every day. If we had the water in front of us, we'd drink it. But we usually don't. And a whole assortment of bad symptoms stems from that.

This may seem paradoxical, but drinking more water can actually make us look and feel slimmer. You know that bloated feeling you get after eating too much salt? Your body must maintain the correct proportion of salt in its cells at all times (a proportion very close to that of seawater); otherwise, all sorts of processes start to misfire. So if you eat a lot of salt, your body holds on to extra water to keep the ratio correct. You feel bloated. By then drinking extra water, you allow your body to flush out the excess salt and still retain the proper balance. Your bloated feeling (and look) goes away.

Drinking plenty of water can also help you lose weight, because one of the ways your body knows it's full is when your stomach expands. Sensing this, your body signals you to stop eating. Your stomach can be expanded with liquid just as easily as it can with food (though this expansion doesn't last as long). If you remember to drink water before and during meals, you will fill up on less food. By the time the liquid is out of your stomach, the food from the meal will have entered your small intestine, which is the second place your body senses that it's full. (This is why you feel fuller fifteen minutes after eating; your small intestine is finally getting the food and is saying, Stop! I got plenty down here.) Overall, you end up eating smaller meals.

Drinking enough water will also help you exercise. The first sign of mild dehydration is fatigue, because sufficient water is needed both to get nutrients to the muscles and brain and to create enough sweat to keep your temperature normal.

Many people who begin walking or running and feel their energy level flag after a mile blame it on their breakfast, but that morning cup of coffee, with no other liquid intake, is really to blame. This is equally true for people at work. They feel that slump at noon and head for the coffeepot, thinking they need caffeine to jump-start their system. In reality, they have the energy in stock; it just isn't being transferred where it's needed. A glass of water will perk them right up, without the serious slump that would come in a few hours when the coffee wore off.

So preventing mild dehydration when exercising or working will keep your spirits and stamina surprisingly high. Even more important, it also prevents the results of more serious dehydration. After fatigue comes loss of appetite, then nausea, headaches, distractedness, and sleepiness. If you see these signs in someone you know, get some water into them right away and see if it makes a difference. Beyond this middle stage lies extreme dehydration, the signs of which are dizziness, muscle spasms, kidney failure, and, in extreme cases, death.

Children and older adults are especially susceptible to dehydration, because their thirst sensors don't work as well. They can easily become dehydrated *before* they ask for a drink, so if you have kids or older parents who live with you, keep pushing the liquids.

Keep pushing the liquids in yourself, too. If exercising hard enough to be pouring sweat, you'll get dehydrated and sluggish before you feel thirsty. You can lose a quart of water through sweat while exercising. Are you really drinking a quart to replace it? Always have a drink before you begin exercising and another when you finish. Unless you are exercising for more than a half hour, or it is extremely hot, you probably won't need additional hydration while exercising.

By having a glass of water when I first wake up, another before and after exercising, and another before each meal, I've already assured myself of getting six glasses a day without even thinking about it. Add in whatever drinks I have with my meals and during the evening, and I hit my goal.

That's one tip for making sure you get your eight glasses in. Here are some more:

- Use a pitcher. Keep it on your desk or counter every day. It can be hard to keep track of how much you drink every day, but if you put a pitcher in front of you in the morning and know it has to be gone by the end of the day, you are more likely to remember. Use an attractive pitcher, maybe pottery or colored glass, to make it feel good every time you pour. Remember, this is all about being good to yourself!
- Try other no-cal drinks. Don't like water? Seltzer has no calories, comes in various flavors, and can be more interesting to drink than plain water. Fruit juices, lemonade, and soft drinks count toward your water intake, but they are loaded with calories, so limit your use of them. Diet sodas are calorie-free, so if they get you off regular sodas or fruit juices, they can make a big difference.

(One recent study found that making no changes in your lifestyle other than switching sugary sodas to diet ones made a difference of five pounds over ten weeks.) If you drink a lot of diet sodas, though, you may be getting dangerously high levels of artificial flavors and sweeteners. Water is a better option. Coffee and tea are diuretics, meaning they cause you to urinate more frequently; count only half their volume toward your water intake. Decaf coffee or tea is fine. Don't count alcohol toward your water intake; and in any case, limit this to one drink at dinner.

- Make it taste good. If you don't like the taste of your tap water, squeeze some lemon in it, use a filter to remove the chlorine and other bad flavors, or drink bottled water.
- Drink a glass in the morning. (After all, you haven't had any water in eight hours!) You'll be amazed at how alert this makes you feel.
- Drink (water) and drive. I spend a lot of downtime in my car, so I always carry a bottle of water with me. In summer, try freezing half-full bottles of water in your freezer. Then fill them up with water and take them with you on any drive. Even in a hot car, they will stay cool all day long.

Drinking enough water is one of the foundations for creating the new you. That's why I've made it one of your new goals in this book. It's free and it's easy—you really have no excuses on this one. And I think you'll find that as you get away from the artificially sweet taste of sodas and fruit punch, you'll start to recognize the crystal-clear, life-giving flavor of a glass of cool, clean water. And you'll never want to go back.

How Much Caffeine Is Okay?

Hey, I'll be the first to admit that I like my morning cup of coffee. Freshly brewed, with a little cream . . . mmm, so good. I wouldn't think to take this pleasure away from you. And it doesn't seem to be necessary: Scientists have been trying to peg various health problems on caffeine for decades, and they haven't been able to make any stick—at moderate levels of consumption, at least.

If you drink only one or two cups of coffee or tea a day, caffeine can be a positive factor in your life. It really does boost your energy and concentration for a short period. People perform slightly better on tests after consuming caffeine. The reason for this is that caffeine is a stimulant; it speeds up your whole system. You breathe faster, your heart circulates blood faster, and you metabolize food slightly faster, so oxygen and nutrients get where they need to go. The downside is that once the caffeine wears off, you get the opposite effect. Everything goes more slowly; you feel a little down and perform a little poorly. You've burned up your energy, and now your body needs to make up for it. If you can make this system work for you by getting that caffeine lift when you need it—before mental or physical exertion—and letting the slump occur when you can most afford it (during the natural afternoon siesta that most people in Mediterranean countries like to take, or at the end of the day), great. But if you find that you are absolutely useless in the afternoons at work, or after dinner when the kids need help with their homework, or that you are not sleeping soundly, then perhaps caffeine is working against you and you need to change your patterns.

Definitely limit yourself to no more than two or three cups a day. More than that may increase your chance of cardiovascular disease and may cause calcium to leach from your bones.

If you are a tea drinker, one nice plus from your habit is the terrific amount of antioxidants in your tea. Antioxidants are nutrients found in fruits and vegetables (tea comes from leaves, after all) that help prevent many, many diseases, including heart disease, stroke, cancer, Alzheimer's, and premature aging. Tea—especially green tea—is packed with antioxidants, and coffee has some, as well.

Walking Wonder

Geri Pittman
SWAN QUARTER, NORTH CAROLINA

Lost 34 pounds

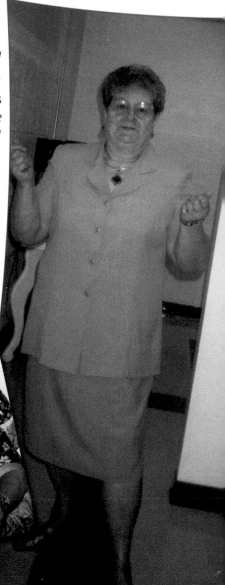

Over the past year, I developed problems with high blood pressure, high cholesterol, acid reflux, and being overweight. I weighed 266 pounds— my most ever. I wanted to do something about my weight problem and get healthy, but I didn't know where to start.

One day, a coworker introduced me to Leslie's Walk Away the Pounds program during our lunch break. I was very excited that this could be done at home. The next day, I started the program. Since then, I have lost five inches through the waistline, several in the arms, and one roll off my stomach. I have lost thirty-four pounds since beginning Weight Watchers and walking with Leslie. I am now at 232 pounds.

I have been averaging from thirty-two to thirty-five miles a week. I try to get in six or seven miles every weekend, and whatever I can fit in during the week. I also use the weighted gloves, ab belt, and some other accessories. I am sixty-eight years young and still work full-time.

I recommend Leslie's program to everyone who tells me how much better I look and asks how I did it. I tell them to stick with a Weight Watchers program, keep a journal, drink lots of water, and exercise with Leslie. I guarantee they will get results.

11. Week 3

GO FOR IT!

Tell me the truth. Are you saying, "Help! I'm *floating* in all this water"? Seriously, though, I bet you're feeling *great*. With two full weeks of walking under your belt, and every one of your cells soaking up that life-giving water, you're starting to get some real rewards. *Feeling* the benefits of walking in the extra energy you have throughout the day is the first reward. *Seeing* the difference in your body shape and muscle tone is the second reward. And *living* this new active, healthy, and *long* life is the ultimate reward! To learn more about the amazing changes taking place in you, read "How Exercise Works," this week's topic for A Little Learning.

This coming week, you get to take your workouts in a whole new direction. You'll increase your daily walks a bit and mix in some hand weights to trigger the upper-body slimming that comes through strength training. Don't be intimidated; strength training is one of those concepts made a lot more complicated than it needs to be. You don't need dumbbells, you don't need fitness machines, and you don't need a pad of paper to keep track of your sets and reps! Once you see how simple it is and how it blasts away fat, you'll be a convert for life.

TOTAL MILES WALKED: 15   USEFUL VIDEOS: *Heart-Healthy Walk*

NEW MILES THIS WEEK: 10   *Super Fat Burning*

A LITTLE LEARNING: How Exercise Works   *Get Up and Get Started*

WALK BOOSTER: Strength Training   *High Calorie Burn*

TAKING STOCK

My accomplishments last week were: _____

_____

_____

_____

My goals for this week are: _____

_____

_____

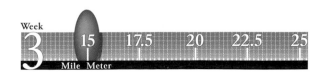

STRENGTH TRAINING

Now to demystify another concept that scares off many women for no good reason. Strength training, or resistance training, is just a fancy term for what you do every time you pick up a baby or a bag of groceries. It's also what you do if you lift weights or do sit-ups. It includes any exercise where your muscles must overcome extra *resistance* from gravity (as with a weight) or from a counterforce (such as pulling against a rubber stretch band). Strength training is not an aerobic exercise, like walking. It involves quick muscle contractions that don't raise your heart rate, so it doesn't deliver much in the way of cardiovascular or mood benefits, but it is the best kind of exercise to increase bone and muscle mass. As I'll explain later in this chapter, the constant contracting and relaxing of muscles during strength training—and the pulling of these muscles against your bones—signals your body to build them even stronger.

Strength training can do wonders for you. The bones of women in their seventies who do strength training are indistinguishable from the bones of women in their thirties who don't. That's right: You can *completely* arrest the bone-loss trend that you hear is "automatic" with old age. Older women who exercise just a few hours per week have 25 percent greater bone density and a 40 percent reduced risk of hip fracture.

Strength training will also do wonders for your looks. You can walk all day, and you'll burn off tons of calories and stay slim, but you won't get that nice muscle definition without strength training. Aerobic exercise makes your muscles work *better*. Strength training makes your muscles *bigger*.

Don't worry about looking like a bodybuilder, or about massive barbells collapsing on top of you. The gentle strength training in my program involves using two-pound hand weights, resistance cords, and rubber stretch bands to get you toned and stylish, not big and beefy. And don't feel compelled to buy all of these. While each works slightly different muscles, you can get the strength training you need from any one of them, or even by using objects you may already have around the house, such as plastic water bottles. See my section on gear in chapter 4 for more information.

If you have been doing a lot of your Walk Diet miles outside so far, I'm going to ask you to do your strength-training days inside. Walking outside is great for the way the changing terrain makes you use lots of different micromuscles, but combining this with weights or belts can throw off your rhythm and increase the risk for twisted ankles and other injuries. Also, some of the moves can't be done properly when moving forward. (Oh, and by the way, you really would look a little funny cruising down the sidewalk, flapping your belt straps like Big Bird. Some things are meant to be done in the privacy of your own home.)

WEEK 3   MONDAY

You're rested. You're fit. You're a three-miler now. But not every day! Don't push yourself too hard today, because we're going to be using the hand weights tomorrow for the first time. Let's do two miles today, but aim to finish in thirty-five minutes—after all, you're not a beginner anymore!

WALK:	2 miles
	35 moderate minutes
	4,000 steps
STRENGTH:	Nothing today

WHEN WILL I WALK TODAY? _____

DID I WALK TODAY? ☐

DID I TAKE MY MULTIVITAMIN? ☐

DID I DRINK MY WATER? ☐

WATER LOG:

1	2	3	4	5	6	7	8
WAKE-UP	BREAKFAST	PREWALK	POSTWALK	LUNCH	ANYTIME	DINNER	ANYTIME

Tip If you carry constant job-related stress in your life, try scheduling your walks first thing in the evening, after you come home. The exercise is like slamming a door on all those issues. You'll make the transition to a relaxed and worry-free night. (Read chapter 22 on stress reduction for explanations why.)

HOW DID I FEEL?

_____

_____

_____

_____

A BEAUTIFUL THING

_____

_____

_____

_____

WEEK 3   TUESDAY

Today is the big day. Are you nervous? Are you trembling in your sneakers? It's time for . . . the dreaded hand weights! Yikes! Run for the hills! Weight lifting! No, seriously, you don't need to be worried about these weights. For one thing, they aren't heavy. They weigh just two pounds each. You've lifted heavier pizzas than that. But two pounds is all it takes to banish flab from your upper body. Best of all, you'll boost the amount of fat you burn. Since this is your first time, do only one mile today. Get used to the weights. As you walk, carry them close to your body for a couple of minutes; then slowly raise them above your head, count to two, and lower them back down. Continue to switch back and forth between the two positions. And never lock your elbows. See page 48 for more specific instructions.

> WALK: 1 mile
>   18 moderate minutes
>   2,000 steps
> STRENGTH: Hand weights

WHEN WILL I WALK TODAY? _____

DID I WALK TODAY? ☐

DID I TAKE MY MULTIVITAMIN? ☐

DID I DRINK MY WATER? ☐

WATER LOG: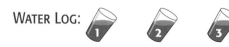

WAKE-UP   BREAKFAST   PREWALK   POSTWALK   LUNCH   ANYTIME   DINNER   ANYTIME

Tip Weighted gloves or balls are better choices for hand weights than dumbbells, which stick out and force you to hold them away from your body. Remember to keep your arms relaxed, yet in control. Large pumping motions are unnecessary. If you find the two-pound weighted balls too heavy, switch to one-pounders. See my section on gear in chapter 4 for more suggestions.

HOW DID I FEEL?

_____

_____

_____

_____

A BEAUTIFUL THING

_____

_____

_____

_____

WEEK 3   WEDNESDAY

Whew! Did yesterday's weights make your arms ache? That burn you feel means your muscles worked hard and then spent the night rebuilding themselves to be stronger and leaner. Good-bye flab, hello elegant arms! Today, we'll take a break from the weights to let your arms recover. Did you ever think that a two-mile walk would feel like such a relief? Try to stick to your thirty-five-minute pace.

WALK:	2 miles
	35 moderate minutes
	4,000 steps
STRENGTH:	Nothing today

WHEN WILL I WALK TODAY? _____

DID I WALK TODAY? ☐

DID I TAKE MY MULTIVITAMIN? ☐

DID I DRINK MY WATER? ☐

WATER LOG: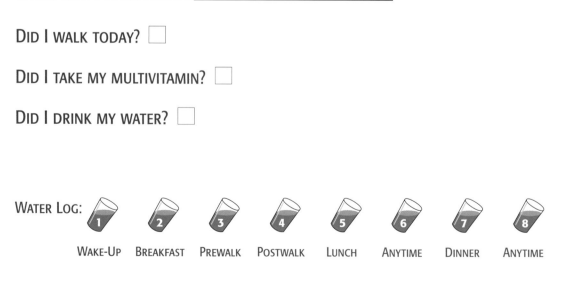

WAKE-UP   BREAKFAST   PREWALK   POSTWALK   LUNCH   ANYTIME   DINNER   ANYTIME

Tip Two-mile walks make calorie-counting supereasy. During an average two-mile walk, you burn a calorie per pound. If you weigh 150 pounds, you've just burned 150 calories. But if you weigh more, say 200 pounds, you can feel even better about yourself because you just burned 50 extra calories!

HOW DID I FEEL?

_____

_____

_____

_____

A BEAUTIFUL THING

_____

_____

_____

_____

Walk Log

Date _____

WEEK 3   THURSDAY

   Good day for unstructured walking—before you begin your big two-day push on Friday and Saturday. Try walking the kids to school or walking to work. If you go grocery shopping, park at the first space you see; don't cruise around waiting for a closer one to open up. If you have a pedometer, clip it on and aim for 7,000 steps. It's a challenge without structured walks!

> WALK: Unstructured
>   7,000 steps all day
> STRENGTH: Nothing today

WHEN WILL I WALK TODAY? _____

DID I WALK TODAY? ☐

DID I TAKE MY MULTIVITAMIN? ☐

DID I DRINK MY WATER? ☐

WATER LOG:

WAKE-UP   BREAKFAST   PREWALK   POSTWALK   LUNCH   ANYTIME   DINNER   ANYTIME

Tip If you'd prefer not to spend any money on weights or other strength-training equipment, there are many creative alternatives you can come up with around the house. Filled plastic 8–16-ounce water bottles work great. Old D-size batteries work fine, too.

How did I feel?

_____

_____

_____

_____

A beautiful thing

_____

_____

_____

_____

Walk Log

WEEK 3 FRIDAY

Time to show what you're made of. Let's do three miles today, followed by two miles with hand weights on Saturday. You're refreshed from yesterday; you're ready to go: let's do it!

WALK:	3 miles
	50 moderate minutes
	6,000 steps
STRENGTH:	Nothing today

WHEN WILL I WALK TODAY? _____

DID I WALK TODAY? ☐

DID I TAKE MY MULTIVITAMIN? ☐

DID I DRINK MY WATER? ☐

WATER LOG:

1	2	3	4	5	6	7	8
WAKE-UP	BREAKFAST	PREWALK	POSTWALK	LUNCH	ANYTIME	DINNER	ANYTIME

Tip Thick rugs can be frustrating to walk on. They feel soft and unsupportive. Linoleum, wood, or thin carpet is ideal; you get all the cushioning you need from a good pair of sneakers.

HOW DID I FEEL?

_____

_____

_____

_____

A BEAUTIFUL THING

_____

_____

_____

_____

Walk Log

Date _____

WEEK 3   SATURDAY

One more day to give it your all. Two miles with hand weights may sound tough, especially on the back of a three-mile day, but just think of the calories vaporizing right off of you. Put everything you've got into this walk, knowing that tomorrow is your free day.

WALK: **2 miles
35 moderate minutes
4,000 steps**
STRENGTH: **Hand weights**

WHEN WILL I WALK TODAY? _____

DID I WALK TODAY? ☐

DID I TAKE MY MULTIVITAMIN? ☐

DID I DRINK MY WATER? ☐

WATER LOG:

WAKE-UP   BREAKFAST   PREWALK   POSTWALK   LUNCH   ANYTIME   DINNER   ANYTIME

Tip If you enjoy the strength training you do in the Walk Diet, you can take strength training to the next level later on with a fitness ball. Those huge balls you've seen are a great way to work a variety of muscles and make it feel like having fun on a playground!

HOW DID I FEEL?

_____

_____

_____

_____

A BEAUTIFUL THING

_____

_____

_____

_____

WEEK 3   SUNDAY

Congratulations! You are halfway through. Now didn't that happen fast? It seems like only yesterday you were worried about that first two-mile walk. Now you look forward to three miles and come out of it more energized than when you started. Time to put your feet up today and treat yourself to a little reward. New jeans? A facial? Dinner in a candlelit restaurant *without* the kids? You pick; just make sure it indulges your spirit.

HOW EXERCISE WORKS

My friend has a convertible sports car. When the weather's nice, he loves to get it out, put the top down, and take it for a spin. It's his way of celebrating what a wonderful, elegant machine it is. Me, I find the most amazing machine to be the one I was born with. To celebrate that, I just take it for a spin.

As machines go, it's hard to beat the body. Your car has only one motor, but your body has millions—every muscle cell is a tiny motor, only instead of using combustion to generate power, it uses chemical reactions. Those chemical reactions release energy that your muscles use to contract and relax, over and over, and make you go.

The fuel for those chemical fires comes from your food. Your muscles take sugar and fat (delivered to them by the blood) and burn them with the help of enzymes and oxygen (also delivered by the blood). Energy is released in the process, along with carbon dioxide and water. Your muscles use the energy, and your blood sweeps away the waste products.

As with a car motor, for this process to work, your body needs fuel (fat or sugar) and oxygen to burn the fuel. It also needs enzymes, which are like little cellular tools. Some chop the fuel into pieces that can be burned; others suck the oxygen out of the blood for the muscle tissue. When you exercise regularly, not only does your body make more muscle tissue; it also makes more enzymes. It wants to give you everything you need to make the job easier. This includes increasing the size of the "pipes" (blood vessels) that carry in fuel and oxygen and carry off waste products. Bigger pipes mean lower blood pressure and less chance of cholesterol sticking to them.

The harder you exercise, the faster this whole process goes. Your muscles need more energy, so they call on the heart to pump faster and the lungs to expand more, allowing you to breathe faster. The result of this hard exercise is that not only do your muscles get what they need but your whole body—including your brain—gets flushed with fresh nutrients. Every time you exercise, you're giving yourself an oil change and a new air filter.

Even your pores get flushed out. The same chemical reactions that supply energy also produce a lot of heat. Your body needs to get rid of that, which is where sweat comes in. To dump heat, you push out little hot-water droplets all over your skin; these evaporate and take the heat with them. Go, sweat, go! Without it, you'd overheat after just a few minutes.

One of the most amazing things about your body is that it uses two different systems for burning fat and sugar. Sugar is stored right in the muscles and can be burned right away, without needing oxygen. This is what happens during the first ninety seconds or so of exercise. If you exert yourself longer than that, your sugar supply in your muscles runs low. Your body thinks, Whoa, I'd better call on the main storage tanks! It starts to liquidate your fat stores and pump that fat through the blood to the muscles, which need it. There, the fat gets burned in a process that requires oxygen. Fat is an amazing energy supply. Nobody—not even marathoners—ever runs out.

If you exercise long or hard enough, though, you get out of breath. Your heart and lungs can only deliver so much oxygen to your muscles. When you start to gasp, you're not getting enough oxygen. And without this oxygen, your muscles can't burn fat at all. They can only burn sugar partway, which results in a waste product called lactic acid accumulating in your muscle. You know the feeling of lactic acid well—it's that burn you feel after working a muscle hard. Your blood will eventually clear the lactic acid out of your muscle, but you'll feel sore the next day.

This is why, if one of your goals in exercising is to burn fat, you want to work out at a pace that gets your heart rate up but doesn't leave you gasping. I bet you're starting to realize why I love walking so much! No other exercise keeps you so perfectly positioned in that level of exertion where your lungs can deliver enough oxygen, fat burns efficiently, and the health benefits pile up. A walker is a fat-burning machine—as wonderful and elegant a machine as was ever created.

Walking Wonder

Betty Nagy
AKRON, OHIO

Lost 83 pounds

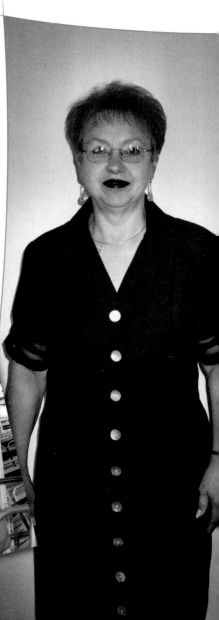

I am fifty-nine years old and have been married for thirty-nine years. My husband and I have five children and ten grandchildren. I started gaining weight thirty years ago after the birth of my third child. I continued to gain and reached my highest weight two years ago, 270 pounds. My cholesterol level and blood pressure were not good, and I was told that I was at risk for diabetes. After another year of being miserable, I finally got serious about weight loss.

In 2002, I started using the Weight Watchers point system and the Walk Away the Pounds *program*. It worked! I found I had more energy than I could ever have imagined. Now I do four miles every morning at 5:00 AM. I have lost eighty-three pounds and have gone from a size twenty-eight to a size fourteen. My blood sugar, cholesterol, and blood pressure are all within the normal range.

I will continue to use Leslie's program as I try to lose another seventeen pounds. I thank God for helping me to have the self-control to get this far, and that will carry me through to my final goal.

12. Week 4

LOVE THYSELF

*T*hree weeks down and three to go! Feeling like a new person? You should be, because you *are* a new person. Your body constantly gets rid of old cells and builds new ones, and yours has been building a whole lot more muscle cells lately. Not only that, but your brain has changed, too. As I mentioned earlier, experts know that twenty-one days is the time it takes to break an old habit and establish a new one. The physical and mental changes that take place during that time make it harder to stop the new habit than to keep doing it. Exercise is your new habit. Your body anticipates it, producing hormones and enzymes designed to take advantage of it when it happens. So you really are transforming, from your head and heart right down to the cellular level. You have sloughed off your old cocoon and a butterfly is beginning to emerge.

Your Walk Booster this week is the key to making your whole new life work. Call it self-acceptance, self-esteem, or whatever you like; it's about falling in love with yourself all over again. If you think this isn't as central to your goals as exercise, then think again! To help get you started on this path, A Little Learning will give you the facts on *real* women in America. You might be surprised!

Keep on walking, and feel good, knowing you are making one of the best choices you can make each mile you go.

TOTAL MILES WALKED: 25	USEFUL VIDEOS: *Heart-Healthy Walk*
NEW MILES THIS WEEK: 12	*Super Fat Burning*
A LITTLE LEARNING: Reality Check	*Walk Away the Pounds for Abs—2-Mile*
WALK BOOSTER: Self-Acceptance	*Walk Away the Pounds for Abs—3-Mile*

TAKING STOCK

My accomplishments last week were: _____

_____

_____

My goals for this week are:_____

_____

_____

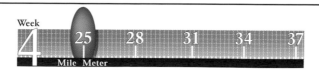

SELF-ACCEPTANCE

Inside many an overweight person is someone who has given up on themselves. No matter the reasons they think they began to gain weight, the truth is that there came a point when, subconsciously, they decided that their body's own needs were less important than the need to put in more hours at work, to drive the kids to ballet lessons, or even just to watch their favorite show with a bag of chips. There is nothing wrong with sacrificing your needs for something else once in awhile, but the danger is that it can steamroll. The more you push yourself aside, the more you forget about yourself. It becomes even easier to push yourself aside the next time. And the more you lose touch with the person inside, the more you suffer the consequences: depression, weight gain, health problems. Then come the dangerous mind traps: "I'm not good enough to deserve careful treatment. Better to concentrate on someone else." "I'm genetically predisposed to be overweight. Nothing can be done." Or worst of all: "I'm going to punish myself for being weak."

Once you hit this point, you are in trouble. Your mind and soul are at odds. You wouldn't treat any of the other important things in your life this way. If your house has a broken furnace, you don't cut off its water supply to punish it. If your daughter struggles in math class, you give her the confidence and support she needs to get better. And heaven knows you've forgiven your husband for all the times he let the grass turn into a jungle! So give yourself the same unconditional love you give others. You absolutely deserve it.

Your Walk Booster for this week is that simple: Toss away negative thinking and give yourself the love and acceptance your soul craves. Don't just make a general commitment to do that this week; assign yourself specific times to work on it. It's your Walk Booster, after all. No matter what your current shape or stamina, as you walk this week, think about the good things you do each day. Then write down three each day. They can be "I walked two miles today!" or "I gave my daughter a big hug before she went to school," or anything else you did of value for yourself or for someone else. As you do this, you'll start to see how we all rely on one another, how we're all a magical part of this magical world. And once you see the magic, *everything* changes.

WEEK 4   MONDAY

Since you rested yesterday, start the week off with another three miles and make this your best fat-burning week yet. As you walk, center your thoughts—and your love—on yourself. Think of the great strides you have made in only three weeks, and how this has reminded you—maybe for the first time since you were a kid—of how much fun it is to move. Let that simple sense of well-being you get from walking begin to spill into the other areas of your life. Are there others you can introduce this happiness to? There's no greater purpose than spreading joy.

WALK:	3 miles
	50 moderate minutes
	6,000 steps
STRENGTH:	Nothing today

WHEN WILL I WALK TODAY? _____

DID I WALK TODAY? ☐

DID I TAKE MY MULTIVITAMIN? ☐

DID I DRINK MY WATER? ☐

WATER LOG: 1   2   3   4   5   6   7   8

WAKE-UP   BREAKFAST   PREWALK   POSTWALK   LUNCH   ANYTIME   DINNER   ANYTIME

Tip On days when you're not strength training, find a beautiful sash or scarf—you know, the one tucked away in the back of your underwear drawer—and tie it around your waist before walking. Use it to remind yourself to tuck that tummy in and to stand up straight while you walk, beautiful!

THREE GOOD THINGS I DID TODAY

_____

_____

_____

_____

A BEAUTIFUL THING

_____

_____

_____

_____

WEEK 4   TUESDAY

Have you read this week's A Little Learning yet? If you have, you know that throughout human history, what's made a woman beautiful is not thinness, but fitness. Thinness is a fairly rare genetic trait; more often, it is the sign of a woman who starves herself. Fitness is the sign of an energized woman actively participating in life. Today, we'll focus that fitness on a new part of your body. The hand weights were great for toning your arms and shoulders; now an ab belt will add strength and tone to your abdominals. Just putting the belt on begins the resistance against your abs that leads to strong, firm muscles. Stretching your arms takes these results through the roof. (For more specific instructions, see page 50.) Remember, the goal is not to make your abdomen disappear; it's to make it smooth and beautifully muscled.

WALK:	2 miles
	34 moderate minutes
	4,000 steps
STRENGTH:	Ab belt

WHEN WILL I WALK TODAY? _____

DID I WALK TODAY? ☐

DID I TAKE MY MULTIVITAMIN? ☐

DID I DRINK MY WATER? ☐

WATER LOG:

WAKE-UP   BREAKFAST   PREWALK   POSTWALK   LUNCH   ANYTIME   DINNER   ANYTIME

Tip Forgiveness is one of the most powerful acts you can practice. Today, try forgiving yourself. We all hold an inner list of grudges against ourselves for things we wished we hadn't done—or had. Holding this regret inside builds tension and unhappiness and doesn't change a single thing in the past. Try letting it all go, truly giving yourself a clean slate to start the rest of your life, and feel the seed of peace that starts to grow inside you at that very moment. It will change your future behavior much more effectively than any amount of self-recrimination will.

THREE GOOD THINGS I DID TODAY

_____

_____

_____

_____

A BEAUTIFUL THING

_____

_____

_____

_____

WEEK 4 WEDNESDAY

How do those abs feel? A little soreness is good; it means you really worked those muscles yesterday. They should start to tighten immediately. Today's an unstructured day. That doesn't mean no walking; it means shake up your routine and get your paces in some other way. Eight thousand steps requires some real exercise, so plan ahead. Call a friend and walk to a café for lunch. Take a stroll after dinner with your husband—when was the last time you did *that*?

> **WALK:**   Unstructured
>   8,000 steps all day
> **STRENGTH:** Nothing today

WHEN WILL I WALK TODAY? _____

DID I WALK TODAY? ☐

DID I TAKE MY MULTIVITAMIN? ☐

DID I DRINK MY WATER? ☐

WATER LOG:

WAKE-UP BREAKFAST PREWALK POSTWALK LUNCH ANYTIME DINNER ANYTIME

Tip If you like to walk outside and need help with motivation, you might want to purchase an amazing invention designed to make you walk every day. Not only does this particular item include unique built-in motivation programs to make walking more fun; it also sends out alarm messages if you try to skip a day. It is called a dog, and you can find one easily.

THREE GOOD THINGS I DID TODAY

_____

_____

_____

_____

A BEAUTIFUL THING

_____

_____

_____

_____

WEEK 4   THURSDAY

Time to get back on that horse—or belt, in this case. Two more miles with the belt should really start to do a number on your abs. If you are predominantly an outdoors walker, this might be a good time to try walking indoors, since combining strength training with the natural instabilities of an outdoor ramble can be awkward.

> WALK: 2 miles
>   34 moderate minutes
>   4,000 steps
> STRENGTH: Ab belt

WHEN WILL I WALK TODAY? _____

DID I WALK TODAY? ☐

DID I TAKE MY MULTIVITAMIN? ☐

DID I DRINK MY WATER? ☐

WATER LOG:

WAKE-UP   BREAKFAST   PREWALK   POSTWALK   LUNCH   ANYTIME   DINNER   ANYTIME

Tip For a mood shifter, try smiling even when you don't feel like it. Researchers who asked two groups of people to perform the same task, half of them smiling and half not, found that the smiling group enjoyed the task more.

THREE GOOD THINGS I DID TODAY

_____

_____

_____

_____

A BEAUTIFUL THING

_____

_____

_____

_____

WEEK 4　FRIDAY

Have you been keeping up with the "beautiful thing" component of the program? What's the most wonderful thing you've noticed so far? My favorite recent beautiful thing was waking, to find my youngest son, Joseph, sleeping at the foot of my bed with his favorite stuffed animal. What a cutie! Beautiful moments can be absolutely anything. It could be the moment when you catch sight of your face in a mirror and think, Hey, I remember that happy person smiling back at me. I can't think of anything more beautiful than that, can you?

WALK:　2 miles
　　　　30 brisk minutes
　　　　4,000 steps
STRENGTH:　Nothing today

WHEN WILL I WALK TODAY? _____

DID I WALK TODAY? ☐

DID I TAKE MY MULTIVITAMIN? ☐

DID I DRINK MY WATER? ☐

WATER LOG:

1	2	3	4	5	6	7	8
WAKE-UP	BREAKFAST	PREWALK	POSTWALK	LUNCH	ANYTIME	DINNER	ANYTIME

Tip Start thinking of your life as a screwball comedy, not a tearjerker. You'll be amazed how this takes the pressure off. Life wasn't meant to be so serious, after all. Once you begin viewing yourself and the other people in your life in the same affectionate way you view sitcom characters, you'll become more forgiving and learn to laugh at things that might have had you steaming before.

THREE GOOD THINGS I DID TODAY

_____

_____

_____

_____

A BEAUTIFUL THING

_____

_____

_____

_____

WEEK 4   SATURDAY

To finish off your own personal love-in this week, let's do three miles with the belt. That should get the old heart fluttering! Wear headphones and blast some music if it helps you keep the pace up. Now, put your hands on your abs. Can you feel the difference? No going back for you. You'll just continue to tone and strengthen—forever! (But if you find yourself moving pianos single-handedly, you might want to ease up on your workouts.)

WALK:	3 miles
	45 brisk minutes
	6,000 steps
STRENGTH:	Ab belt

WHEN WILL I WALK TODAY? _____

DID I WALK TODAY? ☐

DID I TAKE MY MULTIVITAMIN? ☐

DID I DRINK MY WATER? ☐

WATER LOG:

| WAKE-UP | BREAKFAST | PREWALK | POSTWALK | LUNCH | ANYTIME | DINNER | ANYTIME |

Tip For an escape from our culture's prevailing standards of beauty, take yourself to a museum and look at the classical statues, or check out a library book of painting masterpieces. You'll see bodies of all shapes being celebrated. If you were blessed with a full-figured body, think how Rubens would have adored painting you.

THREE GOOD THINGS I DID TODAY

_____

_____

_____

_____

A BEAUTIFUL THING

_____

_____

_____

_____

WEEK 4   SUNDAY

Have you been treating yourself right this week? Finding that sacred center within yourself? True, sometimes it can be hard to find, even when we know it's there, because the noise of the world so easily drowns it out. You aren't alone in this; it isn't even just a modern problem. In the Middle Ages, there were no cars, TVs, or the Internet, yet the Catholic monks still found they had to retreat from the hustle and bustle of daily life in order to see, hear, and feel God in the world around them. They often escaped to monasteries for this purpose—sometimes on islands at the ends of the known world. There they would spend days, weeks, or months in silent contemplation.

You don't have to go to any remote islands or monasteries, but your reward to yourself this week is going to be one those monks would have appreciated. Reward yourself with an hour of silence. You pick the setting. Find the most beautiful church you know and spend an hour in a pew, soaking up the atmosphere. Or try nature's cathedral: Wake up early, step outside, and let yourself watch the sunrise. Don't be in a rush to leave. You can even spend an hour in your very own bathtub—just make sure your family knows they can't disturb you for any reason.

Whatever your hour consists of, it will probably take ten or fifteen minutes for your mind to stop churning. But at some point, the shopping lists, gripes, and pop songs will fall away and you will feel yourself getting in touch with a place of peace we all have within. Your soul will heave one big *aahhhhhh*, and things you thought were bothering you will shrink away. No words adequately describe this place of peace, or the benefits to your life that emanate from it, so you just have to trust me if you've never tried this.

Make yourself do this. It's tempting to think, I know what silence is like and it's not what I need right now. But we *all* need it. And you can't remember the way it invigorates you until you're deep down in it. You may decide that it is a better reward than all the others so far. If so, make sure to do it for yourself at least once a week.

REALITY CHECK

She's thirty-two, a size fourteen, and her days of squeezing into tight jeans are numbered. There's a little wiggle when she walks, a little jiggle when she jumps. There's no hiding her hips, and her abdomen curves out softly.

Recognize this woman? A dropout from the fat farm, maybe? A member of the diet-of-the-month club?

Actually, the person I'm describing was one of the most beautiful women of all time. Marilyn Monroe was her name, and if you didn't read the description above and think, Gorgeous, then count yourself among the many of us who need a reality check. Not so long ago, Marilyn was considered the epitome of female beauty. But if she tried to get a job as an actress or model today? Forget it, honey. Call us when you've lost thirty pounds.

Who knows how our current obsession with thinness started? What matters is knowing that we live in a time that is *not* normal. Standards of beauty have varied wildly throughout different times and cultures; in fact, full-bodied women have been considered beautiful far more often than thin women. We could just as easily live in one of those times, and skinny women like Gwyneth Paltrow would be lying in bed all day and force-feeding themselves bonbons in a desperate attempt to make themselves attractive.

Of course, we don't live in one of those times, and knowing you'd have been considered a bombshell in ancient Greece is little comfort when every magazine and billboard tells you you're overweight. Perhaps we shouldn't blame the ads—their very survival depends on showing us people remarkable enough to make us stop and pay attention—but we sure can blame the beauty and diet industries, which have made a fortune by preying on our insecurities. It's one thing to look at Gwyneth and think Wow, but it's another for books, videos, and magazines to scream at us that we must work out all day, eat nothing but sushi, and get tummy tucks so that we can look like cover models!

Clearly, America needs an attitude adjustment. This starts with learning the difference between two words: *thin* and *fit*. They do not mean the same thing. But ever since Jane Fonda and Olivia Newton-John, we have believed that they do. Even well-meaning scientists have told us for years that to be healthy, we had to be thin. If we weren't, it was because we were too lazy to exercise or too weak-willed to watch our eating.

Now, thank goodness, the pendulum is starting to swing back. A whole new generation of nutritionists is teaching us that a wide range of body types exists, only a few of which were meant to be thin.

But here's where I don't let you off the hook. Only a few people were meant to be thin, but we were *all* meant to be fit. As I said before, our bodies are made to move. Studies are piling up that show it isn't how much you weigh, or even whether you are considered overweight, that determines your health and longevity. It's how much exercise you get—how *fit* you are. Fit full-bodied people live just as long and just as well as fit skinny people. Fit people have good muscle tone, good energy, and the happy dispositions that come with exercise.

In response to these studies, the definition of overweight has changed to accommodate the wide range in healthy body types. A lot of it depends on your individual body type. A woman who is five three and weighs 110 pounds might be just right, but another woman who is the same height and weighs 140 pounds could be perfectly healthy too. See the Body Mass Index chart in the back of this book to determine what your healthy weight should be.

Still not convinced? Then here's a question for you: What is the average dress size in the United States? Six? Eight, maybe? It's actually fourteen. That's right: Normal isn't what you thought it was.

And that's the problem in a nutshell. Our idea of normal and the reality of normal are skewed. That's why your assignment for this week, the Walk Booster that will improve your life on a daily basis, is to shift your mental image of what's normal, healthy, and gorgeous. Skinny is not gorgeous. Skinny is what happens to people when they're malnourished. *Fit* is gorgeous. An active woman with energy, enthusiasm, and confidence who lives life to the hilt—now *that's* gorgeous.

I won't pretend this attitude adjustment will be easy. It won't. You'll be swimming against the current of a powerful media industry bent on convincing you that you need help. You don't. Over the coming weeks, as you put more and more miles under your walking belt and sense how good your new active life makes you feel, I *know* you can break the media's hold on your beliefs. I *know* you can establish a whole new relationship with your body, one based on love and acceptance. I *know* you are on the edge of an exciting transformation.

I know these things because I've seen them happen to hundreds of women just like you. Now it's your turn. I'm excited and grateful to be able to play a role in that, but you are the one doing the hard work. And that's something to look forward to. Nothing feels better than relaxing at the end of a day of hard work, knowing how much you've accomplished. You will achieve great things by the end of these six weeks. The secret: Once you learn to love yourself right now as you are, to give yourself the kind of unconditional love you'd give to a child who needed your help, then everything after that comes easily.

Walking Wonder

Karen Lewis

ALLEN PARK, MICHIGAN

Lost 97 pounds

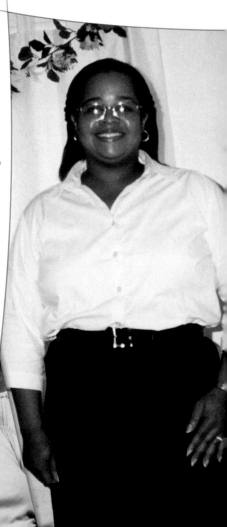

I was a size fourteen and weighed 190 pounds when I got married fourteen years ago. Then I ballooned up to 297 pounds and a size twenty-eight. I felt bad about it all the time and hated to see myself. Then my health really began to suffer. I had high cholesterol, was tired all the time, had constant pain in my knees, and suffered from frequent asthma attacks. My health-care provider said I had to do something and suggested Walk Away the Pounds.

I started watching what I eat and walking away the pounds in September 2001. Leslie shows you how to modify the movements to suit your fitness level. I love to walk now!

Since then, I've lost ninety-seven pounds and many inches. I have so much more energy. I can even run again. I ran a block and cried. You don't know what it's like to be able to do something as simple as run a city block and not be tired. It's amazing. My health has improved, too. The asthma attacks and knee pain are gone, and my cholesterol is under control.

My husband never complained about my weight gain, but I know he's glad to have his old Karen back. My children even told me how proud they are of me. Losing weight has boosted my self-confidence immensely. I see myself and think, Gee, you sure are pretty. I love myself again.

13. Week 5

HIGH GEAR

*L*ook at you. The home stretch and you're still going strong. The finish line is almost in sight—but not quite. This is the point in a race when a marathoner would reach back for that little something extra, so I ask you to do the same. Kick it into high gear. You're close enough to the end that you don't have to worry about burning out. And when you stand on that Week 6 Sunday finish line, you'll be proud knowing that you kept getting better and better.

You're in for some fun this week. The stretch band is the best thing to happen to walking since feet. One simple piece of purple rubber turns your upper body into a state-of-the-art Nautilus machine. The stretch band allows you a wider range of motion than you can get with weights, and adjusting the resistance is as easy as shortening or lengthening your grip. (Using the stretch band isn't quite as obvious as using the weights and belt, so be sure to read the step-by-step instructions for using it on page 51.)

Exercising hard this week, you'll need plenty of rest to keep your energy high, and that's your Walk Booster—lots of good old sack time. Nothing is more important for your well-being. And since you're feeling so well in this fifth week of the new you, what better time to take a look at what could have been. I've told you how an exercise "diet" beats a fad food diet every time, and in A Little Learning, I'll explain *why*. Enjoy learning this for yourself, but also use it to help any friends you might have who are still stuck in the old crash-diet trap.

TOTAL MILES WALKED: 37	**WALK BOOSTER:** Sleep
NEW MILES THIS WEEK: 13	**USEFUL VIDEOS:** *Heart-Healthy Walk*
A LITTLE LEARNING: Why Fad Diets	*Walk Away the Pounds Express—2-Mile*
Don't Work	*Walk Away the Pounds Express—3-Mile*

TAKING STOCK

My accomplishments last week were: _____

_____

My goals for this week are: _____

_____

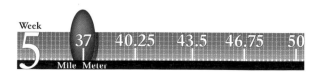

Week
5 | 37 | 40.25 | 43.5 | 46.75 | 50
Mile Meter

SLEEP

The stunning Italian actress Sophia Loren was once asked what the secret was to her radiant beauty. Some special diet? An exotic skin cream? Nope. Sophia said one thing that kept her gorgeous into her sixties and beyond was beauty sleep! Sophia Loren sleeps nine hours a night, plus a one-hour nap after lunch. (She also walks for an hour and a half every day. In fact, Sophia, who drinks a liter and a half of water every day, could be the model for my entire program!)

This week, as you kick it into high gear and raise your metabolism into the stratosphere, keep Sophia Loren in mind. It may sound strange to focus on sleeping during a week devoted to elevating your intensity, but the two actually go hand in hand. Don't feel compelled to sleep ten hours a night, but do make whatever lifestyle changes are necessary to ensure eight quality hours of shut-eye.

For many of us, this requires an adjustment. Immersed in this 24/7 world, it's too easy to think of ourselves as factory machines: Sixteen hours of productivity is good, but twenty would be better. Don't fall for that trap. Good, deep sleep is a vital part of living. While you are snoring away, your body is busy building new antibody cells, adjusting the brain chemicals that regulate mood, reducing stress hormones, and repairing wounds, nerve cells, hurt muscles, and skin. If you don't sleep enough, this stuff doesn't happen, which is why people who don't sleep well have less energy, get more colds, are more irritable, perform poorly on tests, have more accidents and injuries (sleep deprivation causes as many road accidents as drunk driving), and are more likely to be depressed. They also look drained and pale. They even gain weight: Sleeplessness makes people lethargic and chilly, so they consume more food in an attempt to gain energy and warm up, and their sluggish metabolisms convert that extra food to fat.

So I beg you to sleep. You are not lazy when you sleep for eight or nine hours; you are responsible. Do it so you aren't a danger on the road, a crab in the office, or a lump at home. Every time your head hits that pillow, you are embracing life, not shutting it out. Realize that and it becomes a lot easier to fit downtime in. Still, many people have trouble sleeping, even if they do allot the time. If you count yourself among the night owls of the world, here are some tips for turning off during the wee hours. Sweet dreams!

- Exercise every day. (Hah! Didn't think I'd miss that chance, did you?)
- Don't drink caffeine after lunch.
- Don't drink alcohol or smoke before bed. In fact, don't smoke ever.
- Check your medications. Some can affect your sleep.
- Darken your bedroom. And make it is as quiet as possible.
- Lower your stress. Read chapters 21 and 22 on stress reduction for some ideas.

WEEK 5   MONDAY

The stretch band is serious fun, so let's not wait until Tuesday. Do a couple of miles with it today and you'll be hooked. Don't worry about your time too much—getting used to the stretch band moves is enough to concentrate on. (See page 51 for how to use one.)

WALK:	2 miles 34 moderate minutes 4,000 steps
STRENGTH:	Stretch band

WHEN WILL I WALK TODAY? _____

DID I WALK TODAY? ☐

DID I TAKE MY MULTIVITAMIN? ☐

DID I DRINK MY WATER? ☐

HOURS OF SLEEP 🛏 _____

WATER LOG:

1	2	3	4	5	6	7	8
WAKE-UP	BREAKFAST	PREWALK	POSTWALK	LUNCH	ANYTIME	DINNER	ANYTIME

Tip Every walker deserves a foot massage now and then. It is pure heaven for those sore tootsies. Find a local massage therapist and feel those little happy bubbles start to burst in your head as he or she starts massaging. Or get a bedtime rub from your spouse—that's what he's for!—and you'll sleep like a baby.

HOW DID I FEEL?

_____

_____

_____

_____

A BEAUTIFUL THING

_____

_____

_____

_____

WEEK 5   TUESDAY

"I was sore in places I didn't even know I had!" Don't you love that saying? As you rose out of bed this morning, could you relate? If so, thank the built-in flexibility of the stretch band for allowing you to work muscles rarely used. That's why I love the stretch band. That soreness is the muscles complaining. They've been slackers for years, and suddenly they're forced to work! Don't worry; they won't complain for long, once they get used to their new roles. But give them a day off to recover and get ready for Wednesday. Push yourself to do two miles in thirty minutes to keep the calorie burn high.

WALK:	2 miles
	30 brisk minutes
	4,000 steps
STRENGTH:	Nothing today

WHEN WILL I WALK TODAY? _____

DID I WALK TODAY? ☐

DID I TAKE MY MULTIVITAMIN? ☐

DID I DRINK MY WATER? ☐

HOURS OF SLEEP _____

WATER LOG:

1	2	3	4	5	6	7	8
WAKE-UP	BREAKFAST	PREWALK	POSTWALK	LUNCH	ANYTIME	DINNER	ANYTIME

Tip Exercise possibilities are *endless* with the stretch band. Tie one end to your ankle, the other to your chair leg, and get a workout right at your desk while you work!

HOW DID I FEEL?

_____

_____

_____

_____

A BEAUTIFUL THING

_____

_____

_____

_____

Walk Log

WEEK 5 WEDNESDAY

I said high gear, didn't I? Time to put the pedal to the metal and do three miles with the stretch band. As you walk, think, I am a walking machine. And a dancing machine. And a lovin' machine. And . . .

WALK:	3 miles
	45 brisk minutes
	6,000 steps
STRENGTH:	Stretch band

WHEN WILL I WALK TODAY? _____

DID I WALK TODAY? ☐

DID I TAKE MY MULTIVITAMIN? ☐

DID I DRINK MY WATER? ☐

HOURS OF SLEEP _____

WATER LOG:

1	2	3	4	5	6	7	8
WAKE-UP	BREAKFAST	PREWALK	POSTWALK	LUNCH	ANYTIME	DINNER	ANYTIME

Tip People who live in hot climates love my program because they don't have to walk in the blazing heat, but I still encourage the occasional walk outside. It tones slightly different muscles and keeps things interesting. Try walking in the early morning or late evening, when the air is cool and soft.

HOW DID I FEEL?

_____

_____

_____

_____

A BEAUTIFUL THING

_____

_____

_____

_____

WEEK 5   THURSDAY

Day off from indoor walking. If you live near the ocean, stroll a few miles along the beach today. Wear your pedometer; you'll be amazed how the steps add up while you gaze at the waves and the birds. Walking in that soft sand also makes you work harder, so you burn extra calories. Top your walk off with a dip in the sea, and that's what I call a day in paradise! (If you don't live near the sea, take advantage of the natural beauty in your area to create your own day in paradise.)

> WALK: Unstructured
>   9,000 steps all day
> STRENGTH: Nothing today

WHEN WILL I WALK TODAY? _____

DID I WALK TODAY? ☐

DID I TAKE MY MULTIVITAMIN? ☐

DID I DRINK MY WATER? ☐

HOURS OF SLEEP 🛏 _____

WATER LOG:

1	2	3	4	5	6	7	8
WAKE-UP	BREAKFAST	PREWALK	POSTWALK	LUNCH	ANYTIME	DINNER	ANYTIME

Tip Leisure activities that involve walking can pack in a lot of extra miles. Spend the day cruising the booths at a flea market or crafts fair and you won't even notice all the walking.

HOW DID I FEEL?

_____

_____

_____

_____

A BEAUTIFUL THING

_____

_____

_____

_____

WEEK 5   FRIDAY

Let's do three more miles with the stretch band, this time walking fast for the first two miles and slowing down a bit for the final mile. Feel those pounds melting away!

WALK:	3 miles
	30 brisk minutes
	then 20 moderate ones
	6,000 steps
STRENGTH:	Stretch band

WHEN WILL I WALK TODAY? _____

DID I WALK TODAY? ☐

DID I TAKE MY MULTIVITAMIN? ☐

DID I DRINK MY WATER? ☐

HOURS OF SLEEP _____

WATER LOG:

1	2	3	4	5	6	7	8
WAKE-UP	BREAKFAST	PREWALK	POSTWALK	LUNCH	ANYTIME	DINNER	ANYTIME

Tip Don't forget to use the "talk test" while you walk. If you can gab away while walking, you haven't raised your heart rate enough to get the cardiovascular and fat-burning benefits of aerobic exercise. If you are gasping for breath, your heart rate is too high to get the benefits. If you are breathing deeply and can talk in short bursts, you are in that perfect midrange zone.

HOW DID I FEEL?

_____

_____

_____

_____

A BEAUTIFUL THING

_____

_____

_____

_____

WEEK 5   SATURDAY

To finish off your week of high-gear walking, do three miles with the stretch band and keep up the pace. Shoot for forty-five minutes. You are doing wonders! I know you can feel it inside. Forget that arbitrary number on the calendar; where it counts, your body is getting younger, not older.

WALK:	3 miles
	45 brisk minutes
	6,000 steps
STRENGTH:	Stretch band

WHEN WILL I WALK TODAY? _____

DID I WALK TODAY? ☐

DID I TAKE MY MULTIVITAMIN? ☐

DID I DRINK MY WATER? ☐

HOURS OF SLEEP _____

WATER LOG:

1	2	3	4	5	6	7	8
WAKE-UP	BREAKFAST	PREWALK	POSTWALK	LUNCH	ANYTIME	DINNER	ANYTIME

Tip Should you walk when sick? That depends. A mild cold can go away faster if the exercise helps energize your immune system. At the very least, it may make you feel better. But if you have flu or a major illness, your body needs to send all available energy to the immune system. You'll only be taxing it unnecessarily by exercising—and that won't make you well *or* fit.

HOW DID I FEEL?

_____

_____

_____

_____

A BEAUTIFUL THING

_____

_____

_____

_____

WEEK 5   SUNDAY

When was the last day you slept in? I mean *really* slept in—eight o'clock does not count! Today is the perfect day for sleeping in; you've been pushing yourself for a week, so you can afford to be a slug for a few hours and not feel guilty. You've earned it. Open your eyes and think, Aah, Sunday. Notice how good all that quality sleep this week made you feel, how much easier it became to deal with all those things that came flying at you during the week. Grab the paper from the front step and take it back under the covers with you. If you have kids, tell them to call you when breakfast is ready. Better yet, tell them to *bring* you breakfast. (My daughter has become an accomplished cook, and she does this on my birthday now.)

As you lie in bed, think about all the things you have to be thankful for. (Why save this for Thanksgiving? It always feels good.) Think about your support network, about all the people helping you to achieve your goals: friends, family, coworkers, me. Don't forget God! We are all out there rooting for you. The challenges you are undertaking, which may seem insurmountable if you lie awake thinking about them in the middle of the night, are really quite manageable when seen from the cozy comfort of a well-slept-in bed on Sunday morning.

WHY FAD DIETS DON'T WORK

If you've ever tried those weight-loss pills that promise to help you lose something like fifty pounds in ten weeks, you may have noticed the fine print on the back of the package, which says, "For best results, use this product in conjunction with a healthy diet and regular exercise." The little secret they don't want you to know is that the diet and exercise are responsible for all the benefits, not the pill.

The truth about weight loss is incredibly simple, and it can be summed up in two words: *energy balance*! If energy coming in (calories consumed) equals energy going out (calories burned), you stay at the same weight. If you consume more calories than you burn in any given period, your body stores the extra calories as fat. On the other hand (and this is the part I like), if you expend more calories in a day than you consume, your body starts to draw on those same fat reserves to supply the needed energy—you literally burn the fat off your body.

To get a better picture of how your body uses fat, consider squirrels. People love bird feeders, but so do squirrels. Those nice piles of seeds are easy pickings, and squirrels can't resist. In their normal environment, it takes a lot more work to gather food, so when faced with such bounty, squirrels are programmed to grab the seeds and stash them away for a rainy day. This programming is strong enough that it overrides any sort of common sense; it doesn't matter how many hundreds of seed caches a squirrel has, or if he can remember where they all are; as long as that bird seed is available, he's going to keep hitting it.

Our bodies act a lot like those squirrels. For most of human existence, lack of food has been a much more common problem than too much food. So our bodies became very good at grabbing any windfalls and storing them for later. Instead of seed caches, we store the extra food right *on* our bodies—as fat. Fat is an extremely efficient system for storing energy. It works better than a gas tank in a car, better than a battery. We joke about saddlebags on our thighs, but that's what they are—supplies for later in the trip.

The problem arises because, like bird feeders for squirrels, food has become much more abundant than our bodies ever could have imagined. In America, a Whopper or a hot fudge sundae lurks around every corner, just waiting to pounce on us. And our bodies—conditioned by thousands of years of not knowing when our next meal might come—are only too happy to let them.

The way to beat this problem, believe it or not, is to eat *well*. Be good to yourself. If there is an overall message to this book, it is to be good to your body and your body will be good to you. Eating well doesn't mean starvation dieting. Self-denial backfires every time. But eat normal portions of healthy food, without anxiety, and the food traps lose their power over you.

So many people don't see this. Whether choosing the Scarsdale or the grapefruit diet, they are always on the lookout for the same old dream: a magic pill allowing them to eat irresponsibly and still lose weight. To accomplish this, a diet has to cheat the energy-balance equation somehow. And plenty of creative people have come up with ways to cheat.

LOW-CARB DIETS

High-protein, low-carbohydrate diets like Atkins are a favorite of dieters. And no wonder: Talk shows loved to put Dr. Atkins on-screen with a typical lunch of a cheeseburger (hold the bun) and a salad and then have him explain that you can eat this way every meal and lose weight. Bacon and eggs for breakfast, steak and vegetables drenched in butter—who wouldn't be tempted?

Put somebody on the Atkins diet for two weeks and what will happen? They'll lose weight! (Surprised you, didn't I?) But it's mostly water weight, and it may be at the expense of health.

The theory behind low-carb diets is all about sugar. Sugar, the simplest form of carbohydrate and the body's favorite fuel source, gets quickly absorbed by the blood. Eat a candy bar and the sugar is almost immediately transferred to your muscles for energy. Starches such as bread, pasta, and potatoes are just long chains of sugar molecules strung together, so they take only a little longer to break down and be absorbed. Vegetables are also primarily carbohydrates, but they are bound together with fiber and other tough-to-digest material and thus take much longer to break down. Protein also takes longer to digest, and fat takes the longest of all.

When low-carb diets instruct people to eat all the butter, lobster, and bacon they want, the idea is that people will feel sated after a meal and stay that way for many hours while they slowly digest that fat load. When you stay away from carbohydrates, you also avoid quick drops in blood-sugar levels.

One problem with eating almost no carbohydrates is that sugars are essential to good calorie burning. Without sugars, the body can burn only fat. Great, right? Let's eat no carbs and just burn fat all the time! But fat molecules are like big, slow, heavy logs, while sugar molecules burn hot and fast, like kindling. To burn fat completely, you need a steady supply of sugar kindling. Without sugar, the fat molecules burn poorly and leave half-burned residues, known as *ketones*, behind. If you ever tried to make a campfire with wet wood, you get the picture. Ketones are toxic and must be disposed of quickly. To do this, your kidneys start flushing them out of the body. They are washed out in your urine, but in the process, your body loses a lot of water. People who begin low-carb diets are often thrilled to find that they lose several pounds in just a few days, but you know what? All they lost is the water used to flush out the ketones. They become dehydrated, turn into beef jerky, and think they're healthier. (Look for this "jerky" look in people you know who have been on high-protein diets for a long time.)

Over the long term, people on extremely low-carb diets lose weight primarily from boredom: It is no fun to eat a plain hunk of chicken breast every day, cheese or no cheese. You can only eat the mussels straight up for so long before you really miss the linguine. I'm Italian; as far as I'm concerned, life without pasta is no life at all! If you are losing weight because you've lost interest in the foods you're allowed to eat, you've made the wrong choice.

Dr. Atkins did America some real favors. He finally woke us up to the realization that eating low-fat diets very high in sugars and starches actually makes us fatter. He reminded us that some fats are extremely healthy. But while some people have used Atkins or other low-carb diets to eat a balanced mix of carbs, protein, and fat—and have gotten great benefits from their diets—too many others have seen it as a license to eat all the fat they want. And that's where the danger lies.

Problems with irresponsible use of high-protein diets include increased risk of heart disease and stroke; higher rates of prostate, colon, and breast cancer; and deficiencies of fiber and nutrients found in grains. We are not tigers; our systems were not designed to function on a diet of nothing but meat and fat. Eating unnaturally is never a good long-term solution; far better to have a lifestyle that allows you to eat like a real human being and still look and feel great.

RABBIT DIETS

Even worse than tiger diets are rabbit diets—those that cut fat out entirely and give you nothing but a few vegetables and grains to munch on. These diets solve the energy equation by drastically reducing your daily caloric intake. If you eat less, and keep the rest of your lifestyle the same, you should lose weight, right? Alas, our bodies are a bit more complicated than that.

True, if faced with a calorie deficit, our bodies first use up their extra reserves (fat), but if scarce food looks like an ongoing problem, they power down as much as possible to make those remaining energy reserves go as far as they can. Think of animals going into hibernation, shutting down all but the most vital systems.

Faced with a food-restriction diet, your body goes into a minihibernation of its own. Your metabolism—the rate at which your body burns calories—slows down. Sensing that fewer calories are coming in each day, the body slows itself to buy time until the next good source of food comes along. While you don't actually hibernate, you do get sluggish. What's more, you burn fewer calories. Your body cleverly adjusts to your new diet, energy balance is once again achieved, and you stop losing weight.

Eventually, that high-calorie food source comes along—and as we already know, in America such sources are everywhere—and your poor body acts like a bear that just stumbled ravenous from its cave in April. Hello Doritos, good-bye diet. This explains the frustrating yo-yo effect experienced by most people who diet.

Worst of all, when your body takes in fewer calories, it loses lean muscle along with fat. But once you fall off the diet and go back to your original caloric intake, all the new calories are stored as fat until your metabolism catches up again. You are now worse off than when you started: less muscle, more fat, more flab. Because muscle constantly burns calories, while fat just sits there until needed, you will continue to burn fewer calories than you did in the first place, at least until you rebuild your muscle mass. And there is only one way to do that: exercise.

Walking Wonder

Jan Sumner
NEW WILMINGTON, PENNSYLVANIA

Lost 60 pounds

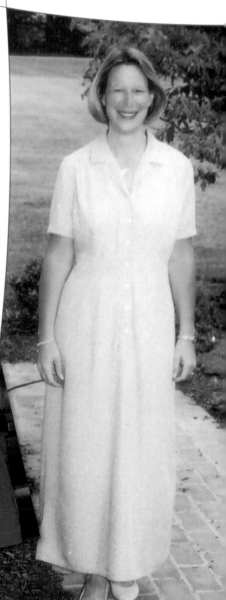

In middle age, I developed bad knees, which made me less mobile and contributed to my weight gain. As I got heavier, I became very self-conscious about exercising in a group situation. Then I discovered Leslie's in-home walking program. It gave me the opportunity to exercise in the privacy of my own home at my own ability level.

When I began, I could barely complete a mile. I continued with that for two weeks before progressing to two miles. Now I can easily do a four-mile walk! Leslie's simple walking steps, coupled with her excitement and enthusiasm, make the program very enjoyable. Unlike some other programs, it's also very easy on the body and joints. I have had two knee surgeries, one a reconstruction, yet I have had no problem completing any of Leslie's workouts. Quite the contrary: They have helped strengthen the muscles around my knees, helping to support the joints.

Leslie's program, combined with healthy eating, has not only helped me to lose sixty pounds but also made me feel better about myself. I have more energy and a much better outlook on life!

14. Week 6

THE POWER OF SPIRIT

*T*he final week of the Walk Diet is the time to put it all together. You've mastered two-mile walks and three-mile walks. You've pumped weights and flexed stretch bands. You know how to keep yourself motivated, hydrated, and animated. This week, mix it up and put the whole program into action. By alternating weights, belts, and stretch bands while you walk, you work every possible muscle and burn fat away from all its hiding spots. (If you don't have all three strength-training helpers, use whatever you do have and try to hit as many muscles as you can.)

The glue that will hold your sixth week together is spirit. We've devoted a lot of time over the past five weeks to thinking about your body. Now let's raise our awareness, forget about the material world for a while, and concentrate on your soul. Your Walk Booster this week tells you to embrace your sacred self. You may have been ignoring it for years, but within all of us gleams a divine spark. Some people have no trouble touching this and knowing it is true. Others find it an effort. That's why A Little Learning will focus on techniques for waking up this part of yourself, in case it needs a little nudge. Once you've got that divine fire inside, everything else comes so much more easily. The exercise, the motivation—they flow as naturally as breathing. In completing this week, you'll find completeness within you.

TOTAL MILES WALKED: 50	USEFUL VIDEOS: *High Calorie Burn*
NEW MILES THIS WEEK: 14	*Super Fat Burning*
A LITTLE LEARNING: Finding the Spark	*Walk Away the Pounds for Abs—3-Mile*
WALK BOOSTER: Walking with Spirit	*Walk Away the Pounds Express—3-Mile*

TAKING STOCK

My accomplishments last week were: ———————————————————

————————————————————————————————————

————————————————————————————————————

My goals for this week are:————————————————————————

————————————————————————————————————

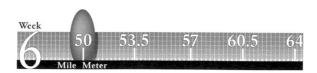

Week
6   50   53.5   57   60.5   64
Mile Meter

WALKING WITH SPIRIT

In Week 4, you accepted yourself as you are. You gave yourself the unconditional love required to build the kind of confident and peaceful core from which all great change emanates. Now, in the final week of the Walk Diet, take that love a step further. Find the sacred in your daily life. Feel in your bones the knowledge that you and every other thing in this universe are part of one and the same creation and are bound together by it. That in itself gives your life great meaning.

What this is really about is extending your acceptance from you to everybody else. We are all related. We all come from the same place. So if you are worthy of love, if *anyone* is worthy of love, then *everyone* is worthy of love. Once you make this leap and accept everyone else as they are, you find some amazing changes happening. Small annoyances become laughable. The victim mentality withers away. No more "Why did he get that promotion instead of me?" or "How can she stay so skinny while eating like a horse?" Instead, you start to think, We are all in this together. How can I help the people around me to realize their dreams and make it clear what I need from them in return? If some of your actions have been driven by fear or sadness, you may find that you see the situation quite differently now.

You have reached the last week of the initial Walk Diet program. If you take just one Walk Booster with you into every day of the rest of your life, let this be the one. When you walk, walk with spirit. Feel the creative love of the universe flowing through you. And when you walk out of the house, take that feeling with you. This is a quiet task, one that can't be counted like so many glasses of water. Protect that feeling like a small bird, warm and safely nestled within you. But know it is there, and draw on it when you need to. You'll never walk the same again.

Date _____

WEEK 6   MONDAY

    Jump-start that divine spark with three vigorous miles of arm-pumping fun. Picture your breath as golden energy, shooting down your lungs, spreading through your chest to your arms and legs, and shining out of your body like a beacon of light.

WALK:	3 miles
	45 brisk minutes
	6,000 steps
STRENGTH:	Hand weights

WHEN WILL I WALK TODAY? _____

DID I WALK TODAY? ☐

DID I TAKE MY MULTIVITAMIN? ☐

DID I DRINK MY WATER? ☐

HOURS OF SLEEP _____

WATER LOG:

1	2	3	4	5	6	7	8
WAKE-UP	BREAKFAST	PREWALK	POSTWALK	LUNCH	ANYTIME	DINNER	ANYTIME

Tip Spiritual and physical energy are like a pair of wings. You need both to fly. If your spirit is down in the dumps, your body will suffer, too. That's why nothing gets me powered up like walking to a CD filled with inspirational music or messages. You can find a nice selection at any bookstore.

HOW DID I FEEL?

_____

_____

_____

_____

A BEAUTIFUL THING

_____

_____

_____

_____

WEEK 6   TUESDAY

No rest for the weary! Keep going hard today, knowing that tomorrow is an unstructured day. Try to finish in forty-five minutes or less. If you have an ab belt, switch to that to give those beautiful abs a workout.

WALK:	3 miles
	45 brisk minutes
	6,000 steps
STRENGTH:	Ab belt

WHEN WILL I WALK TODAY? _____

DID I WALK TODAY? ☐

DID I TAKE MY MULTIVITAMIN? ☐

DID I DRINK MY WATER? ☐

HOURS OF SLEEP _____

WATER LOG:

1	2	3	4	5	6	7	8
WAKE-UP	BREAKFAST	PREWALK	POSTWALK	LUNCH	ANYTIME	DINNER	ANYTIME

Tip If you feel down or sluggish despite your new exercise program, the air might be your problem. Positive ions in the air, created by pollution, TV screens and computer monitors, and cars, cause fatigue, irritation, headaches, and other problems. Negative ions counteract this, improving mood, sleep, and energy. Waterfalls and pine forests are two of the best natural generators of negative ions, but if you don't have one of those nearby you can install a negative ion generator in your own home.

HOW DID I FEEL?

_____

_____

_____

_____

A BEAUTIFUL THING

_____

_____

_____

_____

WEEK 6   WEDNESDAY

One last unstructured walk today before the final three-day push. Some of my favorite unstructured walks involve getting another task done at the same time, such as mowing the lawn with a push mower. Can you think of any more? You'll need to stay active to make your 10,000 steps!

WALK:	Unstructured
	10,000 steps all day
STRENGTH:	Nothing today

WHEN WILL I WALK TODAY? _____

DID I WALK TODAY? ☐

DID I TAKE MY MULTIVITAMIN? ☐

DID I DRINK MY WATER? ☐

HOURS OF SLEEP _____

WATER LOG:

1	2	3	4	5	6	7	8
WAKE-UP	BREAKFAST	PREWALK	POSTWALK	LUNCH	ANYTIME	DINNER	ANYTIME

Tip Ever tried interval walking? Walk fast for three minutes—and I mean fast—then go slowly for five minutes, and then push it again. Increasing your workout for short stretches allows you to intensify your heart rate beyond what you'd be able to maintain over an entire walk and to develop faster than you otherwise would. Interval walking isn't for everybody—but it might be for you.

HOW DID I FEEL?

_____

_____

_____

_____

A BEAUTIFUL THING

_____

_____

_____

_____

WEEK 6   THURSDAY

Back to the stretch band today. You should be feeling the workout this week all over your body. And you should be hearing the thank-yous from every part of your body! Try to do your first two miles in thirty minutes today; then slow down for the final mile.

WALK:	3 miles
	30 brisk minutes, then
	20 moderate ones
	6,000 steps
STRENGTH:	Stretch band

WHEN WILL I WALK TODAY? _____

DID I WALK TODAY? ☐

DID I TAKE MY MULTIVITAMIN? ☐

DID I DRINK MY WATER? ☐

HOURS OF SLEEP _____

WATER LOG:

1	2	3	4	5	6	7	8
WAKE-UP	BREAKFAST	PREWALK	POSTWALK	LUNCH	ANYTIME	DINNER	ANYTIME

Tip Try not to eat for an hour after walking. You'll continue to burn fat for that entire hour—unless you eat!

HOW DID I FEEL?

_____

_____

_____

_____

A BEAUTIFUL THING

_____

_____

_____

_____

WEEK 6　FRIDAY

You need only do a mere two miles with hand weights today. Piece of cake for the fit woman. (Pssst, that's you.)

WALK:	2 miles
	30 brisk minutes
	4,000 steps
STRENGTH:	Hand weights

WHEN WILL I WALK TODAY? _____

DID I WALK TODAY? ☐

DID I TAKE MY MULTIVITAMIN? ☐

DID I DRINK MY WATER? ☐

HOURS OF SLEEP _____

WATER LOG:

1	2	3	4	5	6	7	8
WAKE-UP	BREAKFAST	PREWALK	POSTWALK	LUNCH	ANYTIME	DINNER	ANYTIME

Tip Traveling for work can be one of the biggest challenges to our exercise routine. Fortunately, in-home walking also makes ideal in-room exercising. All you need is this book or a DVD or tape with you. Now that's my kind of room service!

HOW DID I FEEL?

_____

_____

_____

_____

A BEAUTIFUL THING

_____

_____

_____

_____

WEEK 6   SATURDAY

There you are! Right at the very top of the mountain! Go, go, go! You did it!

WALK:	3 miles
	45 brisk minutes
	6,000 steps
STRENGTH:	Ab belt

WHEN WILL I WALK TODAY? _____

DID I WALK TODAY? ☐

DID I TAKE MY MULTIVITAMIN? ☐

DID I DRINK MY WATER? ☐

HOURS OF SLEEP 🛏 _____

WATER LOG:

1	2	3	4	5	6	7	8
WAKE-UP	BREAKFAST	PREWALK	POSTWALK	LUNCH	ANYTIME	DINNER	ANYTIME

Tip Watch out for alcohol. Those empty calories pile up on top of everything you've eaten. A glass of wine has one hundred calories; two a night can wipe out all your walking gains! Plus, alcohol slows down your metabolism. Cut it out entirely, or at least cut your consumption in half, and watch the pounds melt away.

HOW DID I FEEL?

_____

_____

_____

_____

A BEAUTIFUL THING

_____

_____

_____

_____

WEEK 6 SUNDAY

Phew! Sixty-four miles. Hours of strength training. Gallons of water. And now you are at the top of the mountain. Look around, take a deep breath, and enjoy the view. Look at your little trail, stretching away down the mountainside, way down to that teeny-tiny spot in the dark canyon where you started. Can you believe you were ever there? It looks so far away, so distant from you, but believe it. You were there and you climbed your way out, one step at a time. It took a lot of steps—hundreds of thousands, in fact!—but here you are. Now you know you can get to anywhere you want to be. All it takes is belief, dedication, and faith.

I have the perfect reward to commemorate the occasion. Throw a party for yourself! Invite your best friends—the ones who really supported your Walk Diet. Let them bring you presents if they like. This is their chance to let you know how much you mean to them and how proud of you they are. Make sure the party includes something that makes it perfectly clear that you aren't the same person who struggled through that first mile six weeks ago. Go out dancing! Or hike up a real mountain and celebrate up top.

This is also my chance to say thank you. We've been walking together for six weeks. It's been my honor to help you get started on a lifelong path of health and happiness. You can keep walking with me through my videos, books, and Web site, or you can set your own course. Either way, blessings on you. Enjoy the journey, and keep living life to the hilt.

FINDING THE SPARK

Remember six weeks ago when you thought you were buying a weight-loss book? Hah! Little did you know what you were in for! This crazy woman's got you chugging water, looking for butterflies, doing favors for others, and walking with spirit! Can't you just do your steps and be done with it? What's the point?

The point, as I'm sure you've realized by now, is that it's all connected, darling. Your hipbone's connected to your leg bone, your leg bone's connected to your foot bone, and it goes a lot farther than that. Your foot bone's connected to your *brain*, when you get right down to it. Ultimately, your foot bone's connected to *my* foot bone, because when you walk, become more active in life, feel good, and do something nice for me, that makes me feel good and be more active. Then I'm more likely to enjoy my own life and pass the favor on to someone else—or back to you.

This *is* a weight-loss book, but the mistake many people make is to focus on the weight loss in isolation. Weight gain is a symptom of other imbalances in your life. If you do something that addresses only the symptom—like a fad diet or liposuction—then you have done nothing to fix the underlying causes, and the weight gain will return. Fix the factors that caused the problem and the weight gain will disappear on its own. This is why I say, "When you take the focus off weight loss, you get weight loss."

A doctor wouldn't treat you any differently. If you have a dangerous symptom like high blood pressure or cholesterol, he might give you medication to control it immediately, but he knows that unless he gets you exercising and eating better, the problem won't go away. A psychiatrist would say the same thing. Change the person and you change the symptoms.

So yes, this is a weight-loss book. And a fitness book. And a lifestyle book. And a motivation book. And a be-nice-to-others book. And an inspiration book. And a whole lot more besides. But it all comes down to this: All the elements that comprise a healthy life are related, and the point where they all connect is not located in your physical body at all. It's in your soul. When your soul can express itself freely, everything else usually takes care of itself. We all know people who seem completely at peace with themselves. We marvel at how life falls into place for them and wish we could emulate them.

We can. But getting to that point where your soul takes off can be a tricky business. It's one thing to decide intellectually to find that spark in daily life; it's another to feel and live it. But help is at hand. Because it can be so easy to lose touch with your sacred self, people have also come up with many ways to find it again. The following ways are some of my favorites. Not all ways will work for everybody: Some people need to climb Mount Everest to feel spiritual; others are happier volunteering for the Red Cross. Figure out what works for you. But if you find yourself resisting the idea that something magical is at work in the world and that you have a place in that, try *something*; this feeling is too wonderful to miss.

EXERCISE

I won't beat this one to death, since I've been talking about it throughout this book. Exercise not only boosts your mood, it can get you in touch with the spirit moving through all of nature, too. When you work your body, your cells come to life, interacting with the world and taking fresh bits of it into themselves in the form of air, water, and food. This can make you feel powerfully connected, as it should. Native Americans used to go on vision quests, where they fasted and exercised hard for days, until they had divine visions. You don't have to go that far: Your exercise can be an in-home walk; your divine vision can be you in a dress two sizes smaller.

NATURE

Visiting the natural world is one of the best and oldest ways to get a spiritual recharge. When you escape the world of human design, it becomes a lot easier to see other hands at work. Something about the sounds, colors, textures, and patterns of nature soothes the soul. Almost all of us have a park nearby where we can drink in the beauty of lapping waves, shimmering leaves, or soft grass and wide-open sky. It's easy to cut the natural world out of your life altogether, to think it doesn't *really* make a difference, but make yourself go, and more likely than not you'll drive home thinking, I'm really glad I did this.

Nature also helps us get our values in order. What we love in nature is its diversity: the calls of twenty birds at sunrise, the rainbow of fish on a coral reef, the lacework of a snowflake. Remember to apply this value to the human world, too. What makes us beautiful is diversity, not one narrow idea of beauty. Did you ever see an ugly snowflake? Think about this next time it snows.

CHURCH

When was the last time you went to church, or temple, or synagogue? If you were dragged along as a kid, you may have a bad attitude toward church. If so, try it again. When you go by choice, it can be a wholly different experience. The stillness of the pews, the beauty of the architecture, the singing—all help to remind us that there is a higher world interlaced with our mundane one. Even if you are resistant to organized religion, give a church a try. Go with an open mind and no preconceptions and let the spirit take you. Why resist?

VISIT A MONASTERY

Remember those monks I mentioned who would escape from the hubbub of the Middle Ages so they could concentrate on God? They're still out there, in monasteries across the country. And they are only too happy to let you come and visit—no matter what your beliefs. For very little money, they'll give you a Spartan room and some simple food, and you can spend the days walking their gardens and stone paths, reflecting on whatever you wish. Spend the weekend, take a vow of silence, and you will truly feel like a different person when you head back into Monday morning. To find a monastery near you, pick up a copy of the book *Sanctuaries: A Guide to Lodgings in Monasteries, Abbeys, and Retreats.*

MEDITATE

Monks do a fair amount of meditating, but if the idea of hard beds and porridge for dinner doesn't suit you, you can skip the monastery and meditate right at home. Courses in meditation are offered in every city; just look around. The idea behind meditation, and it's a good one, is that our natural state is to be in touch with divine love, but the chatter of the world drowns out this quieter voice. What if there were always birdsong outside your window but you didn't even know it because your son was blasting heavy-metal music upstairs? Get him to turn it off and do his homework, and suddenly that unexpected birdsong comes through loud and clear. Meditation teaches you to turn off the chattering conscious mind so you can hear the spirit song that's been singing in you all along.

CREATE ART

Exploring your creativity is one of the best ways to free yourself from the traps of ego and to get caught up in the give-and-take of life. Whether your thing is guitar, watercolors, or needlepoint, you reach a point where you stop thinking about yourself and get blissfully lost in the process. It's actually pretty close to the feeling you get from a good brisk walk! Great artists talk about the experience of having some power outside themselves take over the creative process, and they just become the hands, whether it's writing a song or a novel, or painting a picture. Pick whatever art form works best for you and let this creative power back in. If you're facing an evening of staring at the tube, get those paints down from the top of the closet and see what you can do (remember: no pressure, no judgment). Then note how satisfied you feel when you go to bed that night.

FALL IN LOVE

We all know that falling in love with another person makes you feel differently about the whole world, not just that person. Suddenly, the flowers are brighter and the coffee tastes better. What happened? You see the relationships between things in a new way; you notice the connections. And that is what finding life's spark is all about. It's no use to *make* yourself fall in love (that usually doesn't work out so well), but try to keep your heart open to love, so that whether it's a new love interest, a friend, or a passionate cause, you are ready to take the plunge.

VOLUNTEER

The greatest way to do sacred work is to serve your fellowman. Seeing that you can make a difference in people's lives, feeling the joy in your own heart that comes with their gratitude, can be as powerful as falling in love. It's one of those few occasions when you don't have to question the value of what you're doing; it's self-evident. Volunteer at a retirement center, a soup kitchen, a day care center, or anywhere else where you know you are needed. At first, you may be volunteering to make yourself feel better, which isn't the real goal, but it doesn't matter. Keep doing it. A day will come when you realize it's about the work after all—and that's when you know you've discovered your inner spirit. (It doesn't even have to be your fellowman. Volunteering at an animal shelter can be an incredibly rewarding experience. Those little fur balls *need* you—and they don't hesitate to show it.)

YOU KNOW YOURSELF

I could go on forever. There are as many ways to feel divine love as there are things to do in the world. Stare at a grain of sand. Make fresh bread. Grow flowers. As I said about meditation, that crystal-clear voice of love is transmitting all the time, through everything and everyone. You just have to figure out how to hear it. You know yourself better than I do, so you get to figure out what works for you. Start today; the only ones who don't find the spark are the ones who don't try.

Walking Wonder

Linda See
STERLING HEIGHTS, MICHIGAN

Lost 42 pounds

I joined Weight Watchers last year after finding myself at the heaviest I had ever been (189 pounds). That weight wouldn't be so bad if I were six feet tall, but at five five I had some work to do. I already had one of Leslie's videos, given to me by the gym teacher at the school where I worked, but I purchased another at the bookstore where I usually shop and got serious about it. Leslie has played a very important part in my weight loss. I have lost forty-two pounds this past year, and I thank God for bringing Leslie into my life. I am now an avid promoter of the program. Lots of ladies from work and church are now fans, thanks to me.

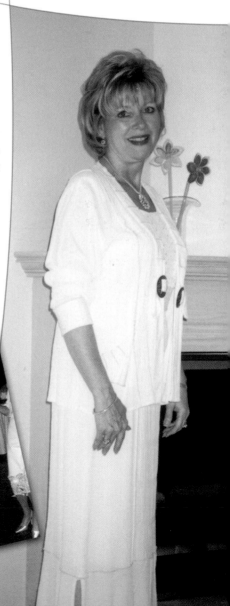

15. Where Do We Go from Here?

Congratulations once again. You are a winner. You set yourself a goal and you achieved it. Walking is now a part of your life. It's a habit, and a great one, just like the other habits built into your new life, like sleeping well, drinking water, respecting yourself, and looking for that rainbow that follows every storm. Maybe when you started, you didn't really expect to be here six weeks later. But that's the beauty of this program—so effective, yet so easy that even those who *don't* expect to succeed usually do.

There are different levels to success. First is starting the program. You did that. Next comes finishing the program. Did that. The third is *maintaining* your fitness routine. That can be a little tougher. Like anything, once the bloom is off the rose and a task becomes old, you can easily lose your enthusiasm. You can even forget where you were when you started the program— how desperately you wanted to make a change and never be in that rut again. To make sure that doesn't happen, I'll offer some suggestions and help you design your own program to keep you walking into the distant future.

For starters, take a good look at the new you. Go back to page 59 and look at the numbers you filled in for yourself six weeks ago. Then fill in your new numbers. If you lost a lot of weight, great, but remember that weight alone can be misleading. Muscle weighs more than fat, so all that lean muscle you built can compensate for a lot of the fat weight you lost. Fluctuations in your menstrual cycle and water retention also can impact weight. More important are your tape measurements; they tell you how much *fat* is gone.

The numbers I care about most are the next ones: blood pressure, cholesterol level, resting heart rate, and glucose (if you have diabetes). If these are down, then you have given yourself the most precious gift of all—longer, better life.

Now look at your before and after pictures. Does the new you have a sparkle in your eye to go with the taut tummy and slender hips? Has your smile broadened? Do you look younger? Those are natural changes that plastic surgery could never duplicate. And there are more to come.

The Hundred Mile Club

If you've reached this point, you are exercising at a very high level. No need to push yourself any harder; the weight-loss and health benefits will keep coming as you maintain your current fitness level. After all, you are burning up to two thousand more calories per week than you were six weeks ago!

For the next three weeks, keep following the workouts in Week 6. After one week, you'll have totaled seventy-eight miles. After two weeks, ninety-two miles. Then, on Thursday of your third week, you will join an elite group: the Hundred Mile Club. That's like walking almost four marathons! (Admittedly, a little slower than some.)

When you join the Hundred Mile Club, let me know so I can post your name on my Web site with the names of the other women who have achieved this milestone of health. That means you're a hard-core walker. That means you're unstoppable! And it means you'd better start keeping track, because we've run out of pages in this book!

The Motivation Station

Knowing that we all suffer from occasional bouts of potatohood, I put together a special chapter (chapter 23) that utilizes the latest science on motivation to keep you maximally engaged with minimal effort. Anytime you feel your resolve weakening, stop by "The Motivation Station" to brush up on your techniques.

Keep a Journal

I love keeping walking journals. They are about so much more than walking. If walking can play a role in all aspects of your life, then a walking journal is the place where your mental, emotional, and physical states come together, where you see the links and reflect on what you need to do to keep yourself on an even keel. Some people like totally blank books, which they can fill in as they see fit. Others prefer more structure, with sections to record their exercising, eating, and emotional state each day. Look around and pick the perfect journal to become your new walking best friend.

FOLLOW MY WALK DIETS ON-LINE

Some people love walking alone. It's peaceful. They can focus. Walking becomes their sacred time. Others are more motivated when they have buddies to share the challenges. I'm aware of both groups, and that's why I offer several Walk Diets a year on my Web site. Just like the Walk Diet you completed in this book, they offer six weeks of guided walks, strength training, and tips. You also get the opportunity to chat with others doing the same Walk Diet, to swap stories with women all over the world. Once you've completed this book, it's the best way to keep me walking with you every day.

VISIT ME

Even better than joining my on-line community is becoming a part of the live community at Studio Fitness in New Castle, Pennsylvania. What better way to celebrate the completion of your first Walk Diet than to spend a week at Studio Fitness and get inspired by my incredible team. You can find out how to contact us in chapter 24, "Let Me Hear from You!"

START A WALKING CLUB

If walking has helped you get your life on track, the best way you can show your gratitude is to turn around and help some others who haven't yet taken the plunge. Many, many of us out there know we should be exercising and *want* to get started, but we don't know how to begin and are just waiting for that first outstretched hand. Invite your friends or coworkers over for a walking party and discover the satisfaction that comes from helping others to realize their dreams.

DON'T FORGET THE REWARDS

Keep being good to yourself as you set out on your own. We all need to remind ourselves every so often that we're special and deserve a little pampering. At this point, you probably need to pamper yourself with a new wardrobe, because all those old clothes are *so* baggy by now. That's my kind of reward—one that feels great, makes a big statement, and reinforces your commitment to staying the course.

POWERWALK

Some time after you've joined the Hundred Mile Club, you may begin to notice a trend you don't like. You are walking just as long and vigorously as ever, but you aren't losing much weight anymore! Classic problem. Plateaus occur when your body gets so fit that it doesn't have to work as hard to do three miles anymore, so you burn fewer calories while exercising. That means you need to figure out how to challenge yourself—and that's what "PowerWalking," my next chapter, is all about.

Walking Wonder

Carol Mortensen

MENTONE, CALIFORNIA

Lost 30 pounds

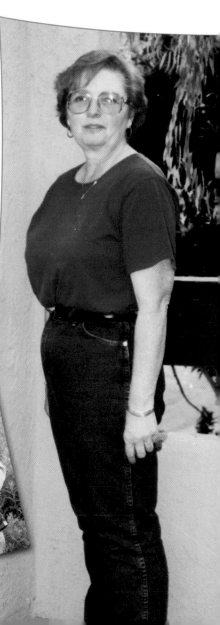

I am fifty-seven years old, and for the past seven years my job has involved lots of travel. Of course, this means much of the time I'm doing nothing but sitting in plane seats and at my desk. I got overweight and developed asthma problems. At times, it was a struggle just carrying my luggage to and from the plane!

Last year, I decided enough was enough and started using Walk Away the Pounds. *I have lost thirty pounds, and the difference in my body shape is amazing! I've lost my saddlebags! My sagging tummy is almost flat!*

I am so excited about the program. When I first started, I thought I would die just doing a one-mile walk. I have now progressed to three-mile walks. I have even started participating in 5K and 10K walks!

In June, I did the Run/Walk over the Coronado Bridge in San Diego. It was one way—uphill. I completed the course in one hour and eight minutes and took only a couple of minutes to recover. I placed 2,595 out of 6,000, eight minutes ahead of the ladies I walked with. I am so happy with my results. I have now signed up to participate in this year's Cancer Three-Day Walk. We will cover twenty miles each day for a total of sixty miles! My pulmonologist has given his approval, and I'm so excited to be participating. Two years ago, I would never have thought it possible that I could or would undertake such an event.

Today, I no longer take any medication for elevated blood pressure, and my asthma is under great control. Best of all, I have been able to do activities with my family this winter that I always dreamed of. I spent Christmas with my son and his family in the Sequoias and went snowshoeing! I loved it, and my grandkids actually tired out before I did.

When people at work ask how I did it, I give credit to Leslie and her program. This is the best tone I've had since my thirties! I feel more energetic and alive than I did when I was twenty years old!

16. PowerWalking: The Advanced Program for Current Walkers

I wrote this book for a number of reasons. One was to reach as many people as possible who thought that fitness was not in the cards for them. Another was to address the multitude of issues that women face in setting up healthy and balanced lives for themselves. Still another reason was to give people who have used my videos for years more guidance on how to design a personalized walking program that will keep them challenged as they get more and more fit. Do the same workout over and over and eventually your body gets locked into one workout and stops progressing. The goal of exercise is to get our bodies to change, but that change is precisely what can leave you on fitness plateaus—levels where you see no additional weight loss even though you are exercising as hard as ever. By exercising, you grow more muscle, improve the strength of your heart and lungs, and create more of the enzymes that take your food and oxygen and transfer it to your muscle. But this means that your body no longer has to work as hard to achieve the same results. A twenty-minute mile might have left you breathless when you started, but now that same mile is a cakewalk. Which only makes sense: You have dropped ten pounds, so there is less of you to move (which takes fewer calories), and your extra enzymes mean your muscles can get the necessary energy to move your body using still fewer calories. You have become an efficient exercise machine—your "miles per gallon" average has gone way up—which is great for your body, but not so good if you are trying to burn more fat. Test yourself: If you are finishing walks and your heart rate is barely elevated, you aren't burning much fat. That may be fine if you have reached your weight goal and just want to maintain your current shape, but if you still hope to shave off a few pounds, you need to step it up to whatever level leaves you working hard but not out of breath. Here are five plans.

PowerWalk 1: Longer Walks

The simplest way to boost your calorie burn is to add a mile to every walk in the six-week program. You achieve perfect fat-burning exertion level for all of those extra miles. You start off with an eleven-mile week, which will be a breeze, and finish with a tough nineteen-mile week, for a total of ninety-five miles in six weeks. Then maintain the nineteen-mile week for a few more weeks. If you want to go this route, you can keep track by posting the list below on your fridge (highest traffic area in my house). Don't forget to keep doing all of your Walk Boosters. If you are using my tapes, try the *4-Mile Super Challenge* on your four-mile days.

WEEK 1

Monday: 2 miles; 4,000 steps
Tuesday: 2 miles; 4,000 steps
Wednesday: 2 miles; 4,000 steps
Thursday: Unstructured; 10,000 steps all day
Friday: 2 miles; 4,000 steps
Saturday: 3 miles; 6,000 steps

WEEK 2

Monday: 3 miles; 6,000 steps
Tuesday: 2 miles; 4,000 steps
Wednesday: Unstructured; 10,000 steps all day
Thursday: 3 miles; 6,000 steps
Friday: 2 miles; 4,000 steps
Saturday: 4 miles; 8,000 steps

WEEK 3

Monday: 3 miles; 6,000 steps
Tuesday: 2 miles w/weights; 4,000 steps
Wednesday: 3 miles; 6,000 steps
Thursday: Unstructured; 10,000 steps all day
Friday: 4 miles; 8,000 steps
Saturday: 3 miles w/weights; 6,000 steps

WEEK 4

Monday: 4 miles; 8,000 steps
Tuesday: 3 miles w/ab belt; 6,000 steps
Wednesday: Unstructured; 10,000 steps all day
Thursday: 3 miles w/ab belt; 6,000 steps
Friday: 3 miles; 6,000 steps
Saturday: 4 miles w/ab belt; 8,000 steps

WEEK 5

Monday: 3 miles w/stretch band; 6,000 steps
Tuesday: 3 miles; 6,000 steps
Wednesday: 4 miles w/stretch band; 8,000 steps
Thursday: Unstructured; 10,000 steps all day
Friday: 4 miles w/stretch band; 8,000 steps
Saturday: 4 miles w/stretch band; 8,000 steps

WEEK 6

Monday: 4 miles w/weights; 8,000 steps
Tuesday: 4 miles w/ab belt; 8,000 steps
Wednesday: Unstructured; 10,000 steps all day
Thursday: 4 miles w/stretch band; 8,000 steps
Friday: 3 miles w/weights; 6,000 steps
Saturday: 4 miles w/ab belt; 8,000 steps

PowerWalk 2: Faster Walks

The chief drawback to PowerWalk 1 is that more miles at the same pace means committing more hours of your week to your fitness program—not something everyone can do. However, you can get all the benefits of those long walks and still have a life by increasing the intensity of your walks. If you're fit, a twenty-minute mile won't burn many calories at all, but a twelve-minute mile will burn lots.

It's easy to find the right level of intensity for yourself; it goes back to my old rule about the "doable challenge." Push yourself to the point where it isn't easy but you still know you can do it—to that midlevel where you are neither gasping nor able to recite the Gettysburg Address with ease. Not only does this provide maximum health and fat-burning benefits; it also keeps exercise fun and rewarding.

If you haven't experimented with interval training yet, now is the time. Interval training involves pushing yourself hard for brief periods during a walk, then falling back to your old pace to recover. Athletes have found that they can improve their performance—and mold their bodies—much more quickly by greatly increasing intensity for brief periods than by gradually increasing it over an entire workout. Your body gets a little taste of what it's capable of and works more quickly to get there.

I build some interval training into all my walking tapes—people don't even realize they're doing it!—but if you are working out on your own, try increasing your pace until you are uncomfortable for a minute, then falling back to your usual pace for three minutes. Then get back to that intense pace for ninety seconds, then back to your standard pace for three more minutes. See if you can eventually get to a point where you alternate equally between your intense walk and your recovery walk.

If walking outside or with a pedometer, you can measure your intensity by how quickly you complete your miles. Follow the standard Walk Diet in this book, but use the following list for time goals. (If you want to use my tapes, the *1-Mile Super Challenge*, *2-Mile Brisk Walk* or *High Calorie Burn*, and *3-Mile Super Fat Burning* all feature fast-paced walks.)

Once you have completed this PowerWalk Diet, continue at the Week 6 pace for three more weeks. At that point, if you sense that you are beginning to plateau again and need to push yourself even harder, then you don't need me—you need an Olympic coach!

WEEK 1	WEEK 4
Monday: 1 mile in 15 minutes	Monday: 3 miles in 42 minutes
Tuesday: 1 mile in 15 minutes	Tuesday: 2 miles w/ab belt in 30 minutes
Wednesday: 1 mile in 15 minutes	Wednesday: Unstructured
Thursday: Unstructured	Thursday: 2 miles w/ab belt in 28 minutes
Friday: 1 mile in 15 minutes	Friday: 2 miles in 28 minutes
Saturday: 2 miles in 30 minutes	Saturday: 3 miles w/ab belt in 42 minutes

WEEK 2	WEEK 5
Monday: 2 miles in 30 minutes	Monday: 2 miles w/stretch band in 28 minutes
Tuesday: 1 mile in 14 minutes	Tuesday: 2 miles in 26 minutes
Wednesday: Unstructured	Wednesday: 3 miles w/stretch band in 42 minutes
Thursday: 2 miles in 30 minutes	Thursday: Unstructured
Friday: 1 mile in 14 minutes	Friday: 3 miles w/stretch band in 42 minutes
Saturday: 3 miles in 45 minutes	Saturday: 3 miles w/stretch band in 42 minutes

WEEK 3	WEEK 6
Monday: 2 miles in 30 minutes	Monday: 3 miles w/weights in 42 minutes
Tuesday: 1 mile w/weights in 15 minutes	Tuesday: 3 miles w/ab belt in 40 minutes
Wednesday: 2 miles in 28 minutes	Wednesday: Unstructured
Thursday: Unstructured	Thursday: 3 miles w/stretch band in 40 minutes
Friday: 3 miles in 45 minutes	Friday: 2 miles w/weights in 26 minutes
Saturday: 2 miles w/weights in 30 minutes	Saturday: 3 miles w/ab belt in 40 minutes

POWERWALK 3: STRONGER WALKS

A superconvenient way to squeeze extra fat burning into your walks is to increase the strength-training component. You can use my existing tapes and can follow the exact Walk Diet laid out in this book, but start with Week 3, where the strength training begins. Instead of two-pound weights, use three- or four-pound ones. If using an ab belt, stretch it a little farther in each direction than you used to, or get stronger resistance cords. With a stretch band, choke up on it, closer to the middle, so that it resists you more with every pull. Don't add strength training to days that don't call for it; it's important to give your muscles recovery periods. (For this reason, if you end up maintaining a Week 6 level for several weeks, take the occasional day off from strength training.)

POWERWALK 4: WALKBLASTER

"When I was your age, I had to walk three miles to school—uphill both ways!" Remember that old joke? Well now, with my WalkBlaster, it really is possible to walk uphill both ways! The WalkBlaster is an inclined, color-coded ramp that burns *more than double* the calories of a regular walk. That'll keep you from plateauing! You can learn more details about the WalkBlaster on my Web site.

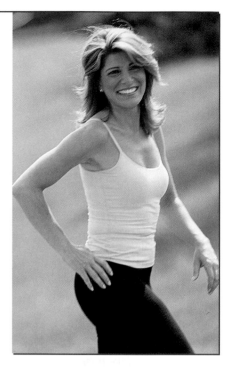

POWERWALK 5: MIX AND MATCH

Hey, it's a free country. Don't feel the need to follow any of the above four plans to the letter. Take whatever appeals to you about each one and combine it. Do longer walks with extra stretch-band sessions. Walk fast *and* long. When you are doing four twelve-minute miles a day while carrying your husband on your back, take a break. Seek therapy.

FOOD, FOOD, FOOD

If you are walking at this terrific level and *still* eating poorly, then you are avoiding the issue. You do not need to burn more calories. You need some healthy ones going in. Not sure what a healthy diet entails? Then take a moment to read chapter 19, "If You Want to Change Your Eating Habits . . ." As with exercise, you'll find that once the subject is demystified, eating healthy food requires no struggle or sacrifice.

Walking Wonder

Jo Fesler
MYRTLE BEACH, SOUTH CAROLINA

Lost 56 pounds

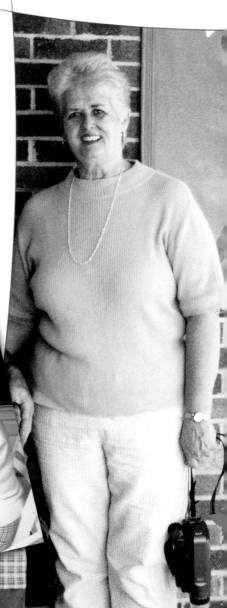

I tried several different methods of losing weight, even my physician's program, but nothing worked for me. It seemed that my willpower was zero. Then I looked over some photographs taken last summer when our grandchildren visited us at the beach. I decided then and there that I did not want my grandchildren to remember me as I looked in those photos. I started to watch what I ate, and lost ten pounds, but I could not do this on my own. As the holidays approached in November, I decided to join Weight Watchers and start a WalkAerobics program.

Along with a coworker, I walked every morning prior to work. We did this for several weeks and then started using Walk Away the Pounds. *Some days we began our workout at 5:30 AM with a four-mile outdoor walk. Some weight started coming off from the change in our eating habits, but the* inches *started coming off because of the exercise we were getting.*

For me, it's been a blessing to lose fifty-six pounds to date. My dress pants have gone from a size twenty-two to a size fourteen in some brands, a size sixteen in others. I still have about twenty-five pounds to lose, and will continue with the change in eating habits and exercise.

I can't speak highly enough for the encouragement Leslie provides. My coworkers and I have become walking commercials for Walk Away the Pounds. *I know for a fact that it really works. It is the commonsense approach to losing weight!*

17. Walking for Two: Pregnancy and the Postpartum Period

Walking and pregnancy go together like . . . well, like mother and child. I know my walking routine made a huge difference during my three pregnancies. I wouldn't have been nearly so active, happy, and healthy without it. I had a different routine with each pregnancy, which had to do with my age and lifestyle. When I got pregnant with Andy, I was in my early twenties, with a fledgling business. Looking back on it now, I'm amazed at what a twenty-something body can do. I was a bouncing superball! I taught advanced aerobics classes—yes, the ones where you leap around and sweat—right up to my due date.

By the time Marie came around, I was thirty. No way was I going to be jumping up and down until my due date this time! Walking was my salvation. It always felt just right, and once again I maintained a full teaching schedule of walking classes until the contractions started.

For Joseph, I was in my mid-thirties. When you are pregnant in your mid-thirties, your body knows to take everything a little slower, and that's what I did. I still kept teaching walking classes—right until my due date—but I taught a few less, and I walked a bit slower. It just felt right. And it must have been right, because I wound up with three of the most beautiful, wonderful kids any mother could ask for.

Being attached at the hip is nothing; for the nine months that your baby is growing inside you, it depends on you for everything—eating, breathing, even working out. Thank goodness we're past the era when doctors put pregnant women in bed and told them to stay there until delivery! Today's obstetricians know that moderate exercise is one of the best ways women can ensure trouble-free pregnancies and healthy babies.

When you realize that your growing fetus is basically an extension of all your systems—cardiovascular, pulmonary, even emotional—it only makes sense that the classic benefits of exercise extend to your little package, too. Some of these pass-through benefits are:

- Improved circulation. By increasing your heart rate and blood flow through your body, you deliver more food, water, and oxygen to the baby.
- Improved immune system. You are your baby's only defense against germs and viruses—not just during pregnancy but for the first few months afterward, as well—-and moderate exercise increases the number of immune cells circulating in your body.
- Better mood. We've spent a lot of time focusing on the fact that exercise puts us in a better mood, and there's every reason to believe that a mother's mood is transferred to her fetus, too. This can be especially nice because of the strange mood swings that sometimes come out of nowhere like small storms while we're pregnant.
- Better birth weight. Low-birth-weight babies are associated with mothers who don't exercise at all.

In addition to the benefits that affect you both, there are some more great pluses for pregnant women:

- Easier deliveries. By increasing the muscles in the hips, pelvis, and back, walking makes you better able to handle the stress of delivery.
- Better support and posture. Strong legs, abs, and back muscles can be key to supporting that extra weight, especially during the last trimester. Let me tell you, carrying thirty pounds cantilevered out over your belly is no easy feat! Most women develop back pain later in their pregnancies because of this. Building up your muscles through walking is perhaps the best way to make sure you can carry the extra weight without slipping into the bad postures that make back pain much worse.
- Better sleep and energy. Sleeping can become sketchy during pregnancy, but walking usually contributes to better z's at night. Even if you are suffering from poor sleep, walking will boost your energy level, refresh you, and make it that much easier to get through the day.
- Less weight gain. You are *supposed* to gain weight while pregnant—twenty-five or thirty pounds is normal and healthy—but walking will help ensure that you don't gain fifty or more. Women who do that are much less likely to return to their prepregnancy weight. And pregnancy is a terrible time to be dieting—your baby needs those nutrients!—so exercise is the sane way to keep your weight gain under control.
- Less morning sickness. Everyone is different. Many of us found that even if we

felt like we wanted to die during our first trimester, once we made ourselves get up and get moving, the nausea subsided. For others, nothing made them want to barf more than a good walk! If this includes you, don't worry; by your second trimester, you'll be feeling *great* and can try exercising again.

HOW TO GET STARTED

One of the nicest parts of my work is hearing from all the joyful women who come to me after discovering that they are pregnant. Helping these women to have healthy pregnancies and to get back in shape afterward really makes me feel good about the role I play in our world.

Some of the pregnant women who are drawn to my program have been active all their lives but are looking for a gentle routine they can use throughout their pregnancies. Other women have never exercised before but know from talking to their doctors that this is the most important time of their lives to get started. A third group of women are the plan-ahead type: They aren't pregnant yet, but hope to be soon and know that exercising before pregnancy is a great way to guarantee a healthy baby.

Whichever category you fall into, the *Walk Away the Pounds* program is perfect for you. Gentle exercise is literally just what the doctor ordered. Of course, check with your doctor first to make sure it *is* what she or he would order. Once you have the okay, you'll want to do a modified version of my program, in this order:

1. Start off with the Week 1 routine. But do it for *two weeks*. Instead of the normal multivitamin, substitute one specially formulated for pregnant women (higher in folic acid, among other things). If this suits you, you can keep doing Week 1 throughout your pregnancy. It's plenty of exercise.

2. After two weeks, if you feel you're ready for a bit more walking, and your doctor says it's okay, move up to the Week 2 routine. The water-drinking Walk Booster is an excellent one to follow during pregnancy: You can have 50 percent more blood circulating through your body in the last trimester, meaning your fluid needs are much higher. You might even want to drink ten glasses—though this means you'll be making a pit stop every ten minutes, since your growing uterus pushes against your bladder. Oh, well; this just makes you look forward to delivery.

3. Do not move beyond the Week 2 routine! Strength training, which normally begins in Week 3, is best saved for after the baby comes—when you'll be lifting an eight-pound weight more times per day than you could ever imagine! Chemical changes in your body during pregnancy actually loosen the connective tissue between your bones and joints. This is what allows your pelvic bones to separate enough to get that baby out. But it also means you are more prone to sprains and pulls. Keep following the Week 2 routine instead. Nine miles a week is all the exercise any pregnant woman needs.

4. As the baby grows, you will probably feel the natural urge to slow down—definitely by your third trimester. This is a good thing. Your body's wisdom is speaking. Listen to it. Stressing your body by overexercising cancels out all the benefits and then some. If you are maintaining a Week 2 pace, drop back to Week 1. If Week 1 feels like too much, switch to half miles, or just exercise on Mondays, Wednesdays, and Fridays. Continue to slow down as needed. Some women enjoy walking right up to their delivery date; others stop before then. Listen to your body and don't do anything that feels wrong.

WARNING SIGNS

Stopping walking any time you don't feel right is always important, but especially so during pregnancy. If you are feeling discomfort, your baby may be stressed, too. Here are some things to keep in mind:

- **Stop any time.** Especially if you are out of breath, dizzy, in pain, or have bleeding or an irregular heartbeat. Your lungs have to work much harder than usual to provide oxygen for two while you are pregnant, so if you are out of breath, so is your baby. (You also aren't burning any fat, of course.) During pregnancy it is more important than ever to stay in that midlevel of exertion, where your heart rate is somewhat raised but you can still talk normally.
- **Drink water** and have a snack a half hour before walking.
- **Don't bounce.** Exercises that cause jerking motions feel very uncomfortable to a pregnant belly and can even weaken the abdominal muscles that support your uterus. Running, dance aerobics, and skydiving are out. Walking, as always, is in, in, in.
- **Warm up.** This is even more important during pregnancy. Warm muscles use oxygen more easily, making it less likely that you'll get out of breath. And you'll have better coordination (a huge problem during pregnancy—believe me!) and lessen your chances of injury.
- **Consider using a sports bra.** Especially during the third trimester, you'll be much more comfortable and will have less chance of suffering a black eye from the "watermelon effect"!
- **Don't strength train.** Save it until after the baby comes. See my discussion earlier in this chapter.
- **Check with your doctor.** Always do this before beginning an exercise program while pregnant, especially if you have a high-risk pregnancy. Some women *shouldn't* exercise while pregnant.

THE POSTPARTUM PERIOD

If you have any doubts that walking is the world's most natural human activity, those doubts will disappear when you have that newborn on your hands.

Generations of sleepy parents have held on to sanity through the lifeline of walking. When *nothing* seems to calm a fussy infant—not nursing, not cooing, not piles of bright toys—a good walk will usually do the trick. There is something in that steady bobbing pace that pacifies us all.

The benefits of walking with your baby go well beyond keeping him or her happy. For starters, it is one of the few exercises you can always do with a newborn. You can't easily squeeze in a set of tennis. You can't run with a baby carrier strapped to you. But walking is a cinch. It allows you to get out and stay in touch with the world, multitasking on exercise, baby soothing, fresh air, and socializing all at once. Using a baby jogger is another great way to get in your walk.

Many women find in-home walking and babies to be a match made in heaven. There are some days when you desperately want to get outside with your kid, and there are other days when it all seems too much—the dressing up, the diaper bag, the changes of clothes. Walking in place in your living room can be a godsend. Your little one can come along for a ride or stay comfortably on the floor next to you. I know a lot of moms who wait until they put their babies down for naps before popping in one of my tapes and getting in two or three miles of undistracted bliss.

Don't expect to lose all that pregnancy weight right away, though. Your body has been through an intense experience, even if the labor went really well, and you need to take things slowly. Wait a month after delivery before trying anything; then double the amount of time spent on each week of my basic Walk Diet. In other words, do Week 1 twice in a row before moving on to Week 2; then do Week 2 for two weeks, and so on. After six months, you should be back to your normal weight. If you aren't back to normal by nine months, make it a priority—the longer you wait, the harder it is to lose!

As your kids get older, you'll find that in-home walking frees you up incredibly. It's the perfect way to navigate those in-between years, when kids are too big for the baby jogger but too small to walk far on their own. Many women find this an especially hard time to squeeze in exercise. You can't leave the house for a jog, but if your kids are napping or playing happily in the other room, nothing is stopping you from taking over the living room. Dad may not be around to put in an hour of child care, but you don't need him. This is a great way to blow off the stress that comes with taking care of small children.

It's also a great way to impart to your kids a superb lifelong habit. Have fun with your walks during this magical time in your life! I firmly believe that by walking while pregnant, by taking your newborn along for the ride, and by letting your toddlers walk whatever distance they can manage, you are giving your kids a huge head start toward a life of health, happiness, and fitness.

Walking Wonder

Robyn Tynan
FENELTON, PENNSYLVANIA

Lost 81 pounds

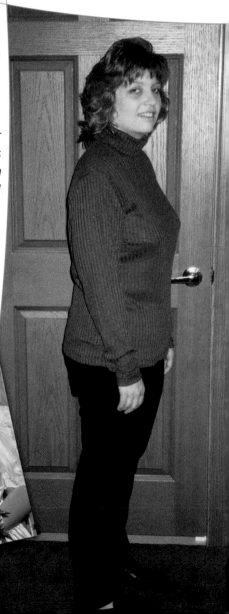

When I became pregnant in December 1999, I weighed 235 pounds. I gained more than forty pounds while pregnant and developed high blood pressure and gestational diabetes. After giving birth to a beautiful baby boy in August 2000, I weighed 258 pounds. I decided that if I wanted to be around to see my son grow up, I had better start living healthier. In January 2001, I joined Weight Watchers.

Weight Watchers strongly suggests that you exercise as part of your program, so in May 2001, I began walking outdoors for fifteen minutes a day, five days a week, but I soon learned that you can't count on weather or a baby to cooperate! I began looking around for a program I could do indoors.

I bought the tape of a well-known fitness personality, but I found the routine too hard to do. Then I came across Leslie's program. From the first mile, her philosophy clicked with me. The exercises were easy to follow, but the results were impressive. The weight began to disappear. Once I had lost fifty pounds, I bought some more tapes for myself as a reward and to vary my routine.

Today, I still walk four to five times per week and am a whole new person. I weigh 177 pounds and have dropped twelve dress sizes! My goal is to lose an additional fifteen pounds. My friends and family have noticed a huge difference in my energy level and attitude about life. I am much healthier than I was. I used to hate exercise, but now I wake up and immediately start thinking about when I will be able to do it. I'm sure these are changes I will continue to incorporate into my (long, healthy) life!

18. Special Considerations for Older Adults

Wendy had been active throughout her life, but in her sixties she began to slow down without even realizing it. Though she ate no differently than she ever had, she began to gain weight. This extra weight made it a little more uncomfortable on those rare occasions when she did try to exercise, so she found herself putting it off. The weight gain continued, and soon the discomfort she felt while exercising crept into her daily life in the form of pain in her ankles, knees, hips, and back. Well, she thought, I guess this is what it's like to get old.

What Wendy experienced is *not* an automatic consequence of aging. Unfortunately, more often than not it is what typically happens in a culture that tries to keep its senior citizens off their feet as much as possible. Amazingly, only one of every five women over the age of fifty exercises regularly. And don't tell me they don't know it's good for them!

But then there is the other story you hear. We all know people in their seventies and eighties who walk, jog, or do other things to stay as active as people half their age. They never seem to grow old. We shake our heads, smile, and say, "How do they do it?" In reality, *they* should be the norm. Our bodies are made to move, and this doesn't stop when we hit a certain age. We are all capable of staying fit into our eighties and beyond. The key, of course, is to use it or lose it.

Even if you lose it, though, you can get it back. Doctors used to think that exercise could slow down the decline that comes with age but that once something was gone, it was gone for good. Now researchers know that older people, even those in their eighties, who begin a gentle exercise program lose weight, rediscover lost energy, rebuild muscle tissue and bone, and suffer far fewer injuries and diseases. They even perform better on memory tests. And their surging happiness level may be the nicest change of all.

Armed with this knowledge, a host of doctors, government agencies, and fitness experts, including me, are working to get the word out: Your senior years may be the most important time of your life to start exercising.

Now, I'm going to ask you a supereasy question. See if you can guess the answer: What exercise is recommended above all others for older adults?

Any ideas? Hunches?

That's right! Walking! How did you guess so easily?

The same things that make walking a great exercise for people of all ages make it ideal for older adults. Other, more vigorous exercises can strain backs and biceps, but no one gets hurt walking. And, unlike yoga or tai chi, older adults already have a good sixty-plus years of experience doing it!

Sure, walking protects older adults from diabetes, heart disease, cancer, and stroke, but the benefits go way beyond that. Normally, women lose about half a pound of muscle a year starting at age forty and replace that with half a pound of fat. This process really speeds up as we age, until by age eighty we have only *one-third* the muscle we had at age forty—plus a lot more fat. Walking helps stop that. When combined with strength training, it completely reverses it.

More muscle means you will be a much better-looking seventy-year-old if you walk regularly, but this isn't about looks. That muscle helps keep you active and independent. It also keeps you from falling. Among older women, hip fractures are one of the most common accidents. But walking reduces the risk of hip fracture by 40 percent for two reasons. First, the regular exercise keeps your muscles strong, joints limber, and balance sharp, so you fall less. Even if you do fall, regular exercise keeps your bones strong so they are less likely to get hurt by the blow. As with muscle, we lose bone mass as we age. The bones of inactive seventy-year-olds look like bird bones instead of mammal bones—fragile and porous. But regular exercise keeps them as strong as those of young adults.

The upshot of these improvements in health is that regular moderate exercise such as walking reduces older adults' chance of death from all causes by an incredible 50 percent. That means quite a few extra years to enjoy the world. To take that cruise like you always wanted. To walk your dog in the park. To enjoy your grandkids. And I do mean *enjoy*, because the extra years you get through walking are *quality* years. Those healthy bones, muscles, and joints mean less pain. Back pain, something almost every older adult feels at one time or another, is caused by stress on the spine and disks of the back. Stronger muscles (in both the back and the stomach) support your weight and take the stress off the back bones. And don't forget that more exercise equals less weight to support in the first place. Which is going to break more: a crane with a huge arm and a small motor and cable, or a crane with a lighter (but stronger) arm and a powerful motor and cable?

Then there is arthritis, the bane of older adults everywhere. No, exercise won't cure your arthritis, but by keeping your joints working, you stay limber and feel the pain from arthritis less. People who exercise regularly feel less pain in general. The exercise releases endorphins in the brain, freeing you from general aches that would have inactive people scrambling for the bottle of Advil.

WALK FOR YOUR MIND

Pain prevention is undoubtedly part of the reason for one of the most amazing powers of exercise: Not only does it keep older adults healthy; it also keeps them happy. I can think of a cluster of reasons for this. Besides the pain prevention, there is disease prevention: People suffering from heart disease or cancer don't tend to be very happy about it. Being independent and able to stay in charge of your own life makes a big difference, too. Being able to stay in charge of your own *mind* may be even more important to your sense of well-being, and, believe it or not, exercise helps with that, too. One study of 350 adults between the ages of fifty-nine and eighty-eight found that those who exercised regularly performed just as well on mental tests six years later, while those who didn't exercise suffered drops in their mental performance. By getting the heart pumping faster, exercise helps to keep a healthy supply of nutrients flowing to the brain. But, as I explained earlier, the biggest factor is that high blood-sugar or stress levels seem to *shrink* our brains as we age, and exercise helps keep these levels steady.

Being mentally sharp, physically independent, and disease- and pain-free all help explain why those who exercise are happier than those who don't. It's never too late to start. Depressed adults between the ages of fifty and seventy-seven who walked for thirty minutes three times per week became free from depression 60 percent of the time—the same percentage of people who were cured by antidepressants such as Prozac! That's why I question doctors who treat older people with depression by shoving bottles of antidepressants at them—pills with dangerous side effects that won't cure these people's health problems. A national program that got everyone over age sixty-five walking would cause a health explosion around this country the likes of which you've never seen—and it might put a few drug companies out of business in the process.

Tips for Getting Started

By now, it should be clear that if you are over sixty-five and haven't exercised in years, the best favor you can possibly do yourself is to get started right away. But you aren't thirty anymore, so there are some things you want to think about before getting started. Follow my suggestions and you can look forward to many years of looking young, feeling great, and living well.

Check with Your Doc

If you have been inactive for a long time, you will definitely want to check with your doctor before starting an exercise program. She or he will be thrilled to hear it but will want to give you a physical and possibly some instructions before you begin. It is all the more essential to do this if you have existing medical conditions. Read my discussion in chapter 4 about various health conditions and exercise, but nothing can substitute for a one-on-one with your own physician.

Go Slowly

It is far more important *that* you start exercising than *how much* you exercise. Especially for older adults, you get most of the benefits from the first stages of effort. One study of seventy-year-olds found that those who exercised at 65 percent of their maximum heart rate got better results (in terms of healthier heart, lower cholesterol, and so on) than those who got their heart rate up to 80 percent of its maximum rate. Exercise always requires your body to do some general maintenance afterward to repair those worn muscles and spent fuel supplies, but older bodies repair themselves much more slowly, so the men in that study who were pushing themselves to the limit weren't giving their bodies adequate time to repair.

Walking is your ticket to building strength and endurance gradually. If the distances in my six-week program seem too much, I encourage you to cut them in half. Then, after six weeks, go back and see if you can do the full program. The important thing is to do only what you can; you get no benefits from exceeding that.

Warm Up, Cool Down

Older muscles are not as flexible, so all the more important to make sure you loosen them up before beginning. A few minutes of very gentle walking gets the blood flowing through the muscles and lubricating them so they will expand and contract smoothly as you walk. Stretching also helps accomplish this. Many people are good about doing their warm-ups, but fewer do the other side of the coin, the cool-down. As muscles burn fuel, they create a by-product called lactic acid. When you feel the "burn" in your muscle while exercising, it's from this lactic acid—it's an *acid*, after all. Cooling down by walking gently for a few minutes at the end, instead of stopping cold, allows your blood to keep flowing through your muscles and removing lactic acid, but this doesn't keep you going hard enough to create fresh lactic acid. The result will be a well-washed muscle and less soreness the next day. In my videos, I always build in gradual starts and finishes for this reason. If you follow them, you're all set. If you walk on your own, try to remember this rule.

DRINK LIKE A FISH

Older adults' thirst sensors don't function perfectly, so they aren't always aware when they are dehydrated. To compound this, because everything moves more slowly as we age, it takes longer for the water we do drink to bubble into our cells. Don't wait until you're thirsty to drink. Drink a nice tall glass of water fifteen minutes before you start exercising to give it plenty of time to work its magic. You'll have more energy when you do start walking. And don't forget to follow my recommendations for drinking water throughout the day.

Walking Wonder

Carol Best
New Castle, Pennsylvania

Lost 68 pounds

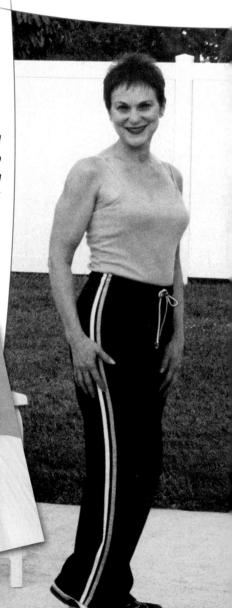

Leslie's program literally saved my life. Like so many of us, I started putting on weight in midlife. As I got heavier, I became less and less mobile. I got to the point where I was in constant discomfort. You think you're dying—and in a way, you are! I knew my life was just going to go down the drain if I didn't do something. I had tried some other exercise programs, but I always found them very hard to do.

Finally, one day I looked at my grandson and realized that if I wanted to see him grow up, I had to change. With him in mind, I worked up the courage to take a class with Leslie. She was incredibly encouraging from moment one, and my doubts melted away. Even though I was badly out of shape, I stayed for the whole hour that first day—which I don't recommend people do! But I was determined, and everyone's energy and enthusiasm were contagious. This made it no problem to keep doing the program.

Now, eight years later, my life has completely turned around. I've lost nearly seventy pounds! I look great and feel so much more optimistic. I sleep better, wake up earlier, and have more energy. Because it is so easy, I think Leslie's program is perfect for the baby boomer generation—those of us who don't want our bodies to take a pounding when we exercise. I have recommended the program to many friends, and even got my eighty-year-old parents started on it! It's made a big difference for them, too—which means they have more time to enjoy their great-grandson!

19. If You Want to Change Your Eating Habits . . .

From the beginning of this book, I promised that you wouldn't have to change your eating habits to follow my program, and it's true. Exercise really is the most important factor in maintaining your weight, health, and optimism. But a funny thing happens to a lot of people after they start exercising. They find that suddenly their body doesn't crave junk food quite so much. Suddenly, the thought of a salad isn't torture. When people get a taste of good health, it feels so good that they want more. They develop a natural craving for healthier fuel. If you are one of those people, then this chapter is for you.

Before we get started, though, I want to say once again that I am not *telling* you what to eat. Food should always be pleasurable. If you are eating a healthy diet because of guilt and self-denial, don't bother, as it won't last. As with walking: Do it because your body wants to, because it makes you feel good.

The message here, as throughout this book, is to *trust your body*. Your body *wants* to be healthy. When you take the focus off weight loss and let your body do the walking it was designed for, the weight loss comes on its own. When you do this, you jump-start the rest of your natural instincts and very often you begin eating a healthier diet without even noticing it: smaller portions, better choices.

I find, however, that many people who develop these healthy urges don't know enough about nutrition to get started. One friend is on a low-fat diet; another is on a low-carb diet. Deciding what diet to choose may seem way too complicated. How are we to know what the right way to eat is?

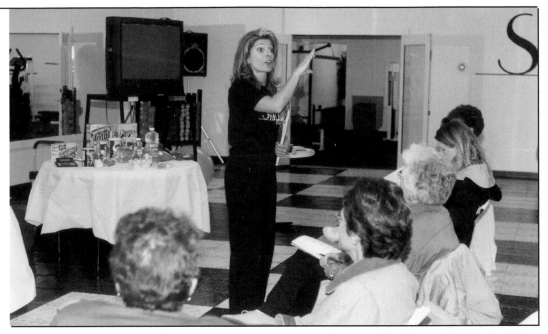
Teaching a nutrition class at Studio Fitness. We try to give our members everything they need for healthy living.

One solution is to follow a responsible diet plan. Weight Watchers has helped millions of people get their eating under control, and I highly recommend their program. Others prefer the low-carb diets, which can work well if you make sure you get a healthy mix of nutrients. All of these diets work well in conjunction with my walking program.

Fortunately, the reality of healthy eating is so simple that you may find you don't need to follow a formal diet at all. In this chapter, I'll explain the basics, then give you ten simple rules to follow that will have you on the road to healthy eating with a minimum of fuss.

Nutrition 101

All food is composed of protein, fat, and carbohydrates (and water). The familiar nutritional information tables on the back of food packages tell us exactly how much of each of these nutrients is in the foods we buy. All three are essential for good health and fulfill different roles in the body, but achieving the right balance among the three can make the difference between a strong, energized body and a fatigued, unhealthy one.

Animals are made up of fat and protein, so when you eat meat or fish, you are consuming fat and protein but no carbohydrates. Plants are made up of mostly carbohydrates, plus small amounts of fat and protein. To get an idea of what each of these nutrients is like, remember that a chicken breast is almost pure protein; sugar, flour, and potatoes are pure carbohydrates; and olive oil, butter, and lard are pure fat.

Proteins are the building blocks that make up your body. Your muscles, skin, and organs are all made up of protein. Getting enough protein each day is essential for children as they grow and for you as you develop bigger muscles through exercise. Good sources of protein are meat, fish, eggs, nuts, seeds, beans, legumes, and soy products such as tofu and veggie burgers.

Carbohydrates are the simplest fuel for your body. If you picture your body being powered by a wood furnace, carbohydrates are the little pieces of kindling you use to get the fire started. They burn fast and hot but burn out quickly. A snack of carbohydrates before a brisk walk can give you an extra burst of energy during the walk.

Carbohydrates differ from one another in how refined, or broken down, they are. Sugars are the most refined form of carbohydrate. Instead of sticks of kindling, they are almost like sawdust. Throw them on your fire and they give off a big burst of heat, but then they're gone and you need to throw on more. This is why when you eat too much sugar, you feel a constant need to eat more. Sugar also doesn't provide you with anything but heat; you get none of the vitamins or other nutrients you get with the other food groups.

Starches, such as rice, potatoes, bread, and corn, are complex carbohydrates. They don't burn up as quickly as sugar, so they provide a more even supply of energy. The more closely they resemble their natural form, the steadier the supply. White rice and white flour have already been broken apart in the factory, so they flame up and flare out just like sugar. Brown rice, whole-wheat flour, and whole corn still have their tough outer shells on, so the body takes longer to digest them, meaning they keep you full longer.

Vegetables are also made up of carbohydrates. But they are bound together with fiber and lots of vitamins, and they take the longest to digest of any carbs. Because of this, they are a key to the super-simple eating rules you'll learn later in this chapter.

If carbs are the sticks of kindling for your fire, fats are the big, slow logs that burn all night. Fats are concentrated forms of calories, packed with energy, so a few go a long way. When you eat fat, it keeps you full for a long time. When your body burns through its carb reserves while exercising—which it does in just a few minutes—it starts burning fat for energy. Fat is a great source of energy, which is why your body packs it on whenever it gets more food than it needs. Fat also cushions your organs and provides a host of other essential functions in the body. *Fat is not the enemy!* Only when you get too much fat do you suffer the health problems too familiar to us: diabetes, heart disease, stroke, cancer, and many others.

So your body needs all three basic nutrients to function at its peak capacity. Problems arise when you get too much or too little of any of the three. Try to get a mix of all three at every meal. This isn't as tough as it sounds. Most dining is built around a natural mix. The classic 1950s "triangular" plate of meat, starch, and vegetable works, as does the sandwich: sliced meat (protein), cheese (fat and protein), veggies (carbs and vitamins), and bread (carbs).

Have you ever tried to do what so many diets recommend and actually count every calorie that goes in your mouth for a week? It's impossible. The portion sizes are never exact, a few ingredients might not match, and you are left with a very rough approximation. This usually turns you into a fussy eater and every dining experience into a math problem instead of a relaxing good time. Instead, follow these ten easy rules and you will cut down on your daily calories, lose additional weight, and get wildly healthy—without even thinking about it.

Ten Rules for Healthy Eating

1. Free Drinks

Calorie-free, that is. As I mentioned in chapter 10, "Water, Water Everywhere," the absolute easiest way to drastically cut calories is to cut all caloric drinks from your diet. Sodas, fruit juices, beer, and wine are equal offenders. If you drink four of these per day, you are stuffing the equivalent of an extra Big Mac down your throat. Worse, they don't even make you feel full; they just make you fat. Switch to diet sodas or unsweetened iced tea (better) or water or sparkling water (best) and watch the pounds fall off.

2. Green Means Go

I can't think of any green food that *isn't* good for you, except maybe that pizza stuck in the back of the fridge for, oh, several months. Green means vegetables, and you can't go wrong: salad, spinach, zucchini, green beans, cucumbers, peas. All are incredibly good for you. When you see green, *go* for it. Eat lots! Not only will you load up on vitamins but you'll also fill up on low-calorie foods. If you go for the greens first, your stomach will fill up before you have a chance to eat so many of the high-calorie meats, cheeses, starches, and sauces. Eating a salad as your first course is a great way to practice this (just make sure you go easy on the dressing, which is very high in calories). If you are one of those people who always leaves vegetables on your plate, you are a prime candidate for the green rule.

3. Brown, Not White

The other color to keep in mind is brown—as in brown rice, whole-wheat bread, and whole-wheat tortillas. These natural forms of grain pack fewer calories per ounce than their white counterparts, have many more vitamins, and take longer to digest. The result? You eat less, feel better, and develop fewer health conditions. The bonus? Once you get used to them, you realize they taste much better, too! Switch from white bread to any multigrain and find out for yourself.

4. All the Veggies, Please

A great place to put all three of the first rules into action is the next time you find yourself in a sandwich shop. You order a sandwich. They ask you what kind of bread you want. Whole-wheat, of course (rule 3). They slap your meat and cheese on. Then they ask if you want any veggies. Say, "All the veggies, please!" (rule 2). You can even say, "Can I get extra veggies on that?" They'll be happy to oblige. And you'll have turned a sandwich into a delicious vitamin machine that keeps you full for hours. For your drink, go for water or unsweetened iced tea (rule 1).

5. Don't Supersize

Here's another great fast-food trick. I have no problem with fast-food restaurants; in my family, we are all so busy that each of us ends up using them occasionally. The trick is to not let the advertising suck you in. If they ask you if you want to alter the size of your meal—and you see how much more you get for only thirty-nine cents—you start thinking that you need that extra food, or that you can't refuse such a great deal. You can, and you should. Bigger is not always better. You don't want your fork supersized. You don't want your cat supersized. Why would you want giant food?

For decades, a cheeseburger and medium fries were what *adults* got for dinner at fast-food joints. Now eight-year-olds are getting burgers and fries that require a flatbed truck to haul them away. You don't need that food to be full. Get yourself the small burger and small fries, or the grilled chicken sandwich or salad. Get a water with that (rule 1) and you're making fast food work for you instead of against you.

A recent study from the Centers for Disease Control and Prevention confirmed that larger portions are the primary culprit in our weight gain. Women's daily calorie intake has jumped from 1,542 in 1971 to 1,877 now—a 22 percent increase. Most of this increase is in carbs—the monster fries and tubs of soda. Even Atkins Nutritionals recently found it necessary to advise its dieters to eat smaller steaks.

6. Don't Skip Breakfast

It's a cliché, but breakfast really is the most important meal of the day. It gives you the energy you need to move, work, and think, and it kicks your metabolism into high gear, so you burn more calories throughout the day. That's right: Skipping breakfast can actually make you *gain* weight. Your body (which has already been fasting for eight hours) misses a meal, thinks food must be unavailable, and powers down so you can survive until that rescue ship shows up! By eating a healthy, full breakfast, you signal to your body that food is plentiful and that it should burn up as many calories as it can.

So many of us skip breakfast, eat a bagel at our desk while we work, and then pig out at dinner to appease the ravenous wolf who's been growling in our tummies for hours. This is the exact opposite of what we should do, because it gives us our fuel when we no longer need it. You wouldn't leave for a car trip with a low tank, run out of gas before the end, push your car the last two miles to your destination, then fill up after you arrived. You fill the tank before you leave, and that's exactly how you should eat each day. Remember one of my favorite sayings: "Eat breakfast like a king, lunch like a queen, and dinner like a pauper."

7. One and Done

Don't bother calorie counting; don't keep track of everything that goes in your mouth—just make the commitment not to go back for more. For a lot of us, that's where the calories start to snowball. One regular serving of lasagna is not a problem, but if we pick at the food while cooking, take seconds at dinner, then kill off the last two bites in the pan when we clear the table, we quietly double our intake. Once you get eating, it feels good to keep going. You don't realize you're full until the food hits your small intestine about fifteen minutes after you eat. By then, it may be too late to prevent overeating. Get the concept of seconds out of your mind *entirely* and you may be shocked at how easy it is to control your eating.

8. Ditch Dessert

I'm sorry, but dessert is doom. It's late in the day, you've probably just eaten your largest meal, you are plenty full, and some well-meaning person plunks an apple pie in front of you—with ice cream. If you partake, you are dumping four or five hundred calories—that's *miles* of walking!—on top of your dinner, with no chance to burn it off that evening. The whole mess gets converted to fat. No way are you going to be able to walk off that kind of habit.

You think you need dessert, but it really is only a habit. Your mouth gets conditioned to anticipate it after dinner. But, like any other habit, if you can stay away from it for three weeks, you'll find the urge has disappeared. (And if you absolutely, positively must have that sweet taste in your mouth, take *one spoonful* of ice cream and walk away. Wait ten minutes. You'll be satisfied.)

9. Split Meals

Have you noticed how meals in restaurants seem as if they're designed to feed the offensive line of the Pittsburgh Steelers? That wasn't true fifteen years ago. Since we have it ingrained in us from childhood to clean our plates, we end up stuffing ourselves whenever we eat out. A great way to stay trim and save money is to split one entrée between two people when dining in a restaurant. Get an appetizer, and then split the entrée. You'll get more interesting flavors and be plenty full. If you absolutely can't pass up the tiramisu, you can split that, too, and still have the bill come in lower than if you'd ordered two entrées.

10. Snack

That's right, one of the best ways to control overeating is to eat *more often*. Am I crazy? Have I bounced one too many hand weights off my head? Not at all. If you eat healthy snacks throughout the day, you simply won't have room to stuff the fattening food in when you do have a full meal. Take the edge off your hunger so it can't take over later on. The key, of course, is to make sure you fill up on *healthy* snacks. Keep foods such as carrot or celery sticks, raw vegetable crudités like red pepper strips and broccoli florets, or fruit within hand's reach all day long. Eat them even when you don't feel so hungry; just grab one whenever you think of it and chew away as you work. You can't possibly gain weight eating these low-cal foods, so eat all you want. You'll find that you eat smaller portions at mealtime and fewer calories overall. Stick to fruits and vegetables for these snack foods; other snack possibilities, such as nuts, are perfectly healthy in small amounts, but they can quickly add up to a ton of calories.

Walking Wonder

Deborah Stuckman
VERONA, PENNSYLVANIA

Lost 85 pounds

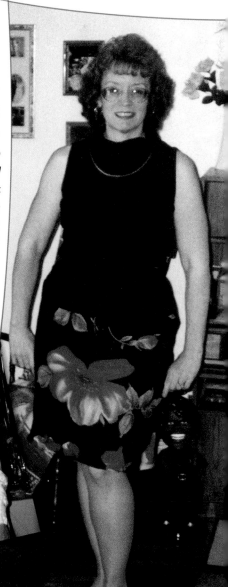

In 1997, I weighed 245 pounds and wore a size twenty. My doctor said I was a candidate for diabetes, which my cousin had died from at age fifty-three. I decided to do something. I switched entirely to fat-free and low-fat food products. At first, it seemed to work. I lost forty-five pounds. But by the time of my daughter's wedding in April 2001, I had put fifteen pounds back on. I didn't understand what was happening.

After the wedding, I went to my doctor. She told me that I should stop concentrating on fat and instead watch my calorie intake. When I did, I couldn't believe it. Sometimes I was consuming seven hundred calories worth of "low-fat" food at lunch alone! I started watching my portion size and tried exercising, but I found it hard to follow the dance routines I tried. Then I discovered Leslie's program while channel surfing and started doing it every other night.

A year later, I weighed 160 pounds! I had to get my mother-of-the-bride dress sized down for Easter! I now wear a size fourteen. I have noticed a change in my muscle tone, as well. I feel so good and so confident. What's nice is that I did it on my own. No pills, no surgeries. When someone tells me they have no willpower, I tell them to quit making excuses. When they say, "Fat cells run in my family," I say, "Mine, too!"

PART IV

MAKING LIFE WORK

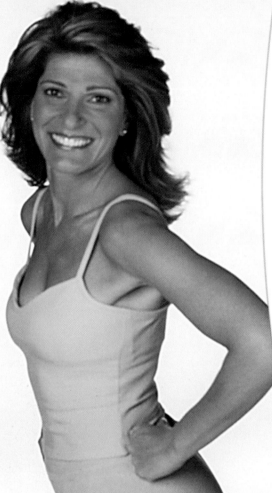

THIS LIFE IS YOURS. TAKE THE POWER TO CHOOSE WHAT YOU WANT TO DO AND DO IT WELL. TAKE THE POWER TO LOVE WHAT YOU WANT IN LIFE AND LOVE IT HONESTLY. TAKE THE POWER TO WALK IN THE FOREST AND BE A PART OF NATURE. TAKE THE POWER TO CONTROL YOUR OWN LIFE. NO ONE ELSE CAN DO IT FOR YOU. TAKE THE POWER TO MAKE YOUR LIFE HAPPY.

—— SUSAN POLIS SCHUTZ

20. The Challenge

Welcome to my favorite part of the book. This is the time when we reach beyond exercise and health issues and get right to the heart of the matter. I can give you the world's easiest and most effective walking plan. I can deliver thrilling pep talks and teach you all about health. I can make you *want* to walk. But if the rest of your life works against this, you will be hard-pressed to make it happen. So many women I talk to tell me how they have a strong desire to get healthy and fit, yet they just don't seem to be able to turn that corner and get started. That's what this part of the book is all about. If you find yourself *thinking* about exercise and weight loss as you rush home from work, driving with your knees while you use a cell phone in one hand and scarf down a burger and fries with the other, then you are a prime candidate for reading these pages.

The challenge for many of us is figuring out how to make life work like it's supposed to. We just feel that something, somehow, is amiss. And I mean we *feel* it. Feel it in the rising stress levels in our bodies. Feel it in the way we never quite get to the important things we want to start because we're struggling so hard to stay above water just dealing with what each day throws at us.

The exercise plan in this book tries to get around this by slipping a bit of walking into your day effortlessly and growing that seed into a full-fledged life of fitness. Many people find that this system is enough to turn the tide. Not only do they get fit but they let this physical transformation shape other parts of their lives. As I said in the beginning, you can harness your newfound energy and use it in ways that go well beyond physical fitness. You can achieve mental and spiritual fitness, too. You can transform your entire life.

Most people find this plan successful, but "most" isn't good enough for me. I want everybody to succeed. And I know that the ones who don't succeed usually have incredible stress and motivation issues in their lives. No wonder: Today's women face more demands by far than our female ancestors did. I'll talk about that in the next couple of chapters. If you find yourself missing too many days of walking—if you've started the plan a couple of times and bailed out halfway through—don't get discouraged. Instead, slide over to these chapters and see if some simple changes can start making life—and fitness—work for you. Use these chapters however you want, but here's a rough game plan to follow.

LET ME SHARE MY STRESS WITH YOU

My life could easily bury me under stress, so I've learned a lot about how to head stress off at the pass or defuse it when it comes. Despite the pressures and responsibilities I face, I think I manage to lead a very normal life. See what you think. Maybe my strategies will give you some ideas. At the very least, you'll know you're not alone.

LEARN A THING OR TWO ABOUT STRESS

Too many people think stress is just an unavoidable nuisance. They live with it like they would houseflies. But if stress is a pest, it is the kind that carries deadly diseases and health conditions, such as high blood pressure, stroke, heart disease, ulcers, depression, premature aging, and many more. Stress is one of the most serious problems we face in our society. Once you learn the facts, you'll be motivated to eliminate stress from your life as much as possible—and I'll give you the tools to do that.

LET'S TALK MOTIVATION

Experts have changed their tune on motivation quite a bit. The idea that most people can be taught to succeed by releasing some hidden, heroic willpower is out. Good thing, because this implies that if you can't access your inner superwoman, you are some kind of wimp. What experts have found is that most of us fail if we exist in an environment conducive to failure, and most of us succeed when put in a no-fail environment. I'll teach you how to set up such an environment for *whatever* it is you want to do, whether that's getting fit or running for president.

I hope you will use these tools to do great things with your life. You know how hard it is to get out of bad lifestyle habits and become fit. So many women have been fighting that battle all their lives. We tend to get down on ourselves about this. "Gosh, if I can't even make myself exercise, I'll never be able to accomplish anything more significant in the world." But, as I'm sure you realize if you've completed the six-week Walk Diet by now, that first step is always the hardest. Once you get momentum, accomplishments snowball. Instead of thinking, I can't even do this; therefore I can't do anything, you should be thinking, If I can do this, I can do anything. Making life work—your entire life, and the lives of others—is no harder than making yourself get off that couch and go. Use the techniques in the following chapters to reduce stressful distractions that sap your energy and focus, to motivate yourself by creating an environment that maximizes effectiveness while minimizing effort, and to take the world by storm.

21. Stress Is My Life

I hear it all the time: "Leslie, you must love your life. You have the perfect job. You just walk and get paid to do it. Somebody shoots a video of you walking, you release the video, and you're done. How easy is that?" Well, I do love my life, but is it easy? No! I chose a life for myself that includes a very, very full plate, day in and day out. It can be a fun and rewarding life, but the stress could easily consume me. I have to keep my perspective at all times to make sure that I run my life, not the other way around. Over the years, I think I've become pretty good at being all the people I need to be: mother, wife, daughter, businesswoman, housekeeper, fitness coach, cook, video star, community member, and friend, not to mention self!

Still think I've got it easy? That once the cameras stop rolling, I plop down on a couch, eat grapes, and lift my feet when the cleaning lady comes by? Hah! I invite you to accompany me on a typical day in the Life of Leslie. Hold on tight. We're going for a ride.

Up and at 'em! It's 6:29 AM and my alarm is about to go off, but I'm already up. Every weekday, I set my alarm for 6:30, and every day, I wake just before it buzzes. Maybe I'm overly responsible. Maybe I just can't stand that sound. (And by the way, if this were a weekend, I certainly wouldn't be rising at 6:30. I can sleep in with the best of them. I love having a tight structure to my weekdays, and I love breaking that structure on weekends. That's what weekends are for! That's what your Walk Diet Sundays are for.) I leave my husband snoozing and head downstairs.

Don't you love the peace of a house first thing in the morning, before anyone else is up? It's my favorite time of day. The stillness is great for slowly gathering your thoughts. First thing I do is pour a glass of water and drink it down. Just like that, my day is off to a positive, healthy start.

You're going to laugh about what I do next. Almost every weekday, I pop in a load of laundry right away. Call me crazy, but there is something comforting about the sound of a dryer first thing in the morning. There is a softness to the sound in my still-sleeping household.

Then it's time for coffee—another great way to gather your thoughts. Sometimes I check E-mail and phone messages as I sip, but usually I go straight to the calendar on the fridge and see what the kids have going that day. Who's buying lunch, or who's taking lunch. (Why can't they just decide one way or the other?) Who has after-school activities. Focusing on this now, knowing what's coming at me ahead of time and being able to plan a little order for the day, is a key to keeping unwanted surprises from stressing me out. I try to get lunches made and backpacks ready by the time Joseph, my eight-year-old, and Marie, my twelve-year-old, stumble down for breakfast at 7:00 AM.

My kids are good breakfast eaters. They learned this healthy habit from me. Marie makes her own breakfast now. Without being the biggest nag in the world, I try to get a little protein into Joseph every morning: an egg, toast with peanut butter, or at least cold cereal with milk.

Sometime after breakfast finishes up, it happens: *Boom!* The explosion! Good-bye peaceful morning, good-bye orderly day. I'd be lying if I told you that the nice head

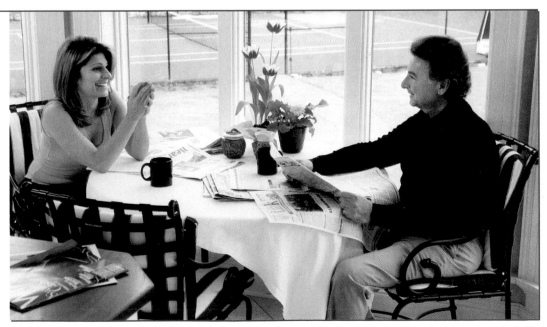

Enjoying a rare moment of morning quiet with Joe. Coffee, the paper, good company—does it get any better?

start I get on my day results in a well-executed march to the car with all items neatly accounted for. No. Usually, with about fifteen minutes until we have to leave for school, I'm putting out fires on all fronts. "Joseph, where are your socks? What happened to that note from your teacher?" Duke, our golden retriever, has gotten loose from Marie on his morning walk again and is doing his best to wake up our neighbor, a doctor who gets in late and needs his sleep. It is chaos, but I wouldn't have it any other way. I have a big appetite for life, and this family energy, stressful as it can be, is a big part of life. Whether you let it irritate you or you learn to love it for what it is goes a long way toward determining whether it results in unhealthy stress in your body or not. Is this stress going to affect my life a week, a month, a year from now? Almost never. Is it something I can laugh about someday? Almost always.

I'll let you in on a secret for gauging the chaos level of my morning. If you happen to be at my kids' school when I drop them off, and I am still in my favorite black robe, the chaos is particularly intense that day. Yes, I have been known not to make it out of the robe in time. I just throw my coat over it and head out. However, the robe has holes in it that Duke chewed when he was a puppy (he just loved that thing!), and lately the holes have been getting bigger. Now I'm starting to get caught on things as I go by. Someday I will fail to show for a meeting because I'm snagged in a tree somewhere.

With my robe becoming more and more of a stay-at-home item, I really do try to get changed into exercise clothes *before* I leave the house each morning. Not

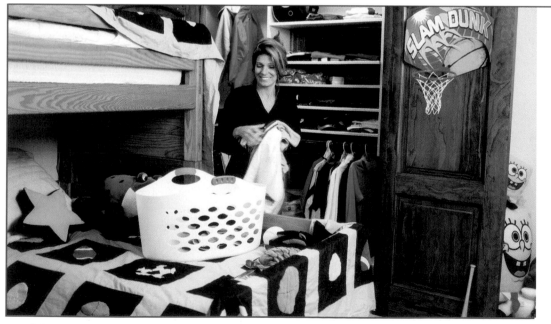

Caught! Doing laundry in my old black robe. At least Joseph had his room straightened up that day.

only does this save me time and energy but it helps ensure that the first thing I'm going to do after I drop off the kids is exercise. May as well—I already have the clothes on! Try putting on your exercise clothes first thing and see if that doesn't get you in the workout mood.

Of course, if I'm scheduled to teach at the studio that morning, I don't have any choice. One great, great benefit about the life I've chosen is that it forces me to do the thing that I love. Being "forced" to do something you love may sound funny, but often that's what it takes. With the demands upon us, we are usually only too willing to sacrifice the things we love to other obligations. If at all possible, I recommend making your love and your life one and the same.

If I'm not teaching that morning, I return home and exercise with one of my tapes. Yep, I use them, too! At this stage of my life, I always exercise in the morning. With my business growing and my family having a full evening schedule, I know that if I don't work out early, I probably won't. Years ago, when my business was young and I didn't have kids, I taught evening classes and exercised then. Fun memories, but I wouldn't go back.

I should mention that when my kids were young, I took *full* advantage of having my mom, sisters, brother, good friends, and other family members close by. They were an incredible support network. I don't know how I would have done it without them. I think the lack of close family nearby during the early child-raising years is a major source of stress for many modern families. You never truly appreciate your mother until you have a two-year-old on your hands!

By nine o'clock, the kids are at school, I'm done with my workout, I've showered, and I'm raring to go. The double tonic of a healthy breakfast and morning exercise has me energized and enthusiastic. Both of which I'll need to be, because my first wave of daily stressors is about to hit.

I have a home office. When not teaching at Studio Fitness, I try to work from there as much as possible. I get much more accomplished, and with less agitation. I'm a homebody. It's been such a blessing that my work has allowed me to travel both throughout this country and many others and meet all sorts of wonderful people, but my favorite moments are right here in my snug home. From here, I can handle all my correspondence and go over scheduling and finances for my business. In addition to the logistics for classes at Studio Fitness and for my schedule of filming and media events, there are endless tasks necessary to keep a business running properly. Taxes, health insurance, payroll. If you're a small business owner, you know what I'm talking about! I currently have thirty-five employees on-site, not including our teams of Walk Leaders across the country. Then there are the people I work with at QVC, *Woman's Day*, Goodtimes Entertainment—and, of course, Warner Books! All are excellent and rewarding relationships for me, but all require a piece of the pie that is Leslie's Day. As you can see, if I wasn't careful, there wouldn't be any pie left for me!

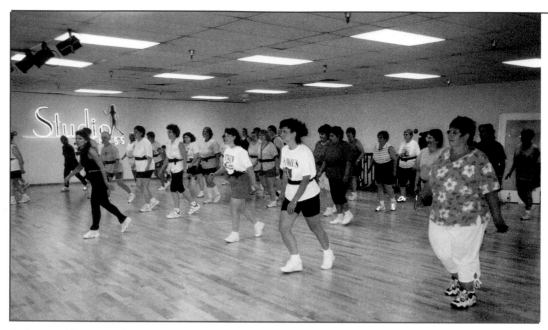
Doing our thing at Studio Fitness. Come join us anytime!

But I am careful. At least now I am. I wasn't always. I used to slip into the trap of being available to anyone at any time. When the media called, I always dropped everything for an interview on the spot. The folks at QVC have been a dream to work with, and we are almost always able to schedule my appearances months in advance, but every now and then they get a last-minute gap in their schedule and ask me to fill in, sometimes only a couple of days ahead of time. They never pressured me to do it, but in the old days I would put my life on hold and catch the next flight to Philadelphia to do the show.

Now I've become much better about managing my time. If I can squeeze in the show, I do it. If I can't, I let the opportunity pass. I let a lot of opportunities pass now, and I'm much happier for it. My stress level stays low. There is a lot of work out there, and we're all tempted to run after it, but at some point you have to stop and ask yourself whom and what you're running for. The answer may change your priorities.

So over the years I've learned to say no. Business opportunities have come up where I stood to make a lot of money, but they involved people using my image in ways that made me uncomfortable. I said no.

I don't obsess over money. I can't think of a better way to send your stress hormones racing than to focus on the bottom line all the time. My experience has been that business is a series of relationships between groups of people, and if you concentrate on making the relationships work out, the money will be there for you to continue to accomplish what you need to accomplish in this world.

So much for my home-office life. Studio days raise the stress bar to the next level. Thirty-five staff members, hundreds of customers. It's kind of a giant version of the postbreakfast explosion. When you have that many variables mixed into your day, things go wrong. Such is life. It's how you deal with it that makes the difference.

Recently, we lost power just as a large class was about to start. No lights, no audio equipment—no problem! We hit the parking lot for some outdoor walking tips. You should have seen the thirty-five of us cruising up and down the lanes of parked cars!

The events that have the most potential to stress me out, the ones that really get me, are when somebody comes to Studio Fitness for the first time and doesn't have a good experience. It takes tremendous bravery to walk alone through a health club's door for the first time, and I hate to see even one of these brave souls turned off by the experience. When it happens, I could stew about it, which would not help at all. Instead, I try to embrace it as an opportunity to correct a mistake. Sometimes the best relationships in life start off on the wrong foot. By making the effort to get beyond that, you wind up with stronger bonds than if nothing had gone wrong in the first place. That's a secret to success I'd like to spread around. Never dwell on past mistakes or disappointments. Move on to plan B—even if you don't have one yet!

If my life doesn't sound hectic enough yet, let's talk about the days when I do have to travel. I've gotten pretty good about clumping all my travel demands into a

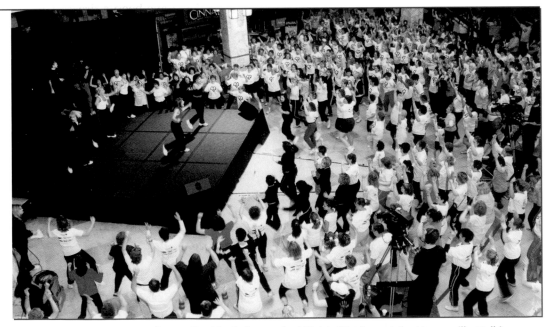

Filming the world's largest indoor walk with Florine Mark of Weight Watchers at the Monroeville Mall in Pennsylvania. That'll get you charged up!

couple of days a month, but oh, what those days involve! Of course, they couldn't happen at all if I didn't know I could count on my wonderful husband, Joe, to be there for the kids. Knowing he's there, I can concentrate on shooting my new tapes and QVC appearances.

I film in New York, and the crew is always setting up by seven o'clock in the morning, getting ready for what we all know will be a twelve-hour day. The equipment is so expensive that once it's up and running, we want to get as much as possible out of it. Usually, we finish a new shoot in two days. This is a tiny fraction of the time that most new videos take, and it is because I insist on not choreographing the video. We keep the foundations of fitness intact, and then we just shoot one take. Why put a lot of pressure on yourself to make it look too perfect? That just makes it harder for real people to follow at home, anyway. Sometimes we can shoot three related videos in a single day. Believe me, video companies appreciate this!

These days are grueling, but invigorating, too. I get a real charge out of the energy of everyone involved and from learning new things. I certainly never pictured myself in front of a camera when I began teaching aerobics in church basements twenty-five years ago!

About the only thing that gets me more charged up than shooting videos is going live on TV. Live TV, with millions watching, is about as scary as it gets! Before airtime, my stress hormones start racing, but it's the good kind of stress, the kind that helps me deliver a peak performance. A half hour after filming, the adrenaline is all burned up, and that's when I can come in for a controlled crash landing.

I love the intensity of those days, but I'm glad they aren't that frequent. It's the mix of filming days, event days, studio days, and home days that is the real secret to my longevity. That mix keeps everything fresh. Twenty-five years, and no burnout so far. Think I can go another twenty-five? I'll keep you posted.

As I said, the home days are the ones that feel most like the "real me." By late afternoon, I'm ready to shut down and make the transition to the kids coming home. They're always famished when they walk in the door, so I try to have healthy snacks ready for them. I'm a softy; I'll still peel and cut up an apple for my son, rather than making him do it. I just know it's a lot more likely to go down that way. Raw veggies with healthy dips are constants in our house. (And yes, chips and cookies are semiregular visitors, too. Hey, life is balance.) Because my kids have such active after-school schedules, I've found one thing that keeps us all sane and functioning is to have an early dinner—maybe around five o'clock—and *then* head out for softball, voice lessons, and the rest of the jumble of activities that make up today's kids' lives. That allows us to maintain the peace and structure of family dinners without making the kids cut back on their schedules.

Actually, we *have* cut back a little. There was a point when we were slipping

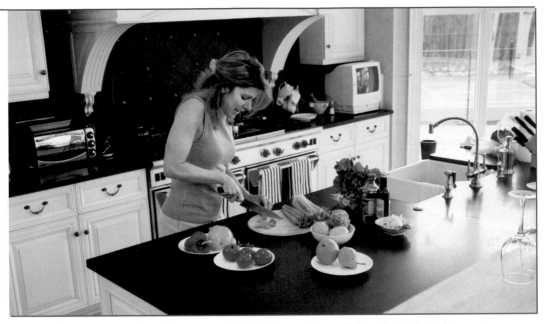

Starting to cook an early family dinner. Lots of fresh fruits, veggies, and olive oil—it's the Italian way!

toward "overscheduled child" syndrome. Fortunately, we recognized that and pulled back. If you find yourself hitting the drive-through window for dinner most nights, if you feel like you never see your kids and never talk, then think about pulling back. It made a big difference for us.

Part of the problem is the crazy number of school sports offered these days. With football, softball, swimming, lacrosse, and on and on, there are no longer enough kids to stock all the teams, so coaches aggressively *recruit* kids to their sport, and let kids double and triple up. When I watched one of my son's friends strip off his football uniform at halftime, race over to the marching band for the halftime performance, and then charge back to the team afterward carrying his tuba like a giant football, I saw dangerous stress rearing its head.

Your kids are going to want to do as much as possible, and the last thing you should do is forcibly stop them—you know that backfires—but help them to keep it under control. Make sure family life isn't threatened by basketball practice. Just like you, your kids need unstructured days for spiritual rejuvenation. Trust your deep feelings on this matter, as on all others—they're almost always right!

Once the activities wind down, in the evenings, we're just your basic American family—and does it get any better than that? We do homework, read, watch a little TV. We play games and tease one another. I must admit that I follow Sophia Loren's lead—I *struggle* to stay up until ten o'clock! I need my full eight hours plus to feel healthy, happy, and energetic the next day. When my kids were younger and needed me to lie in bed with them, I confess that half the time I never made it out of the bed. Today, if I want to indulge myself and watch *Larry King Live* or the *Late Show with David Letterman*, I actually set the *alarm*, go to sleep, and then wake up to watch!

That's a rarity, however. Usually, I just let myself fall asleep, amazed that this full and rewarding life has come to be. I drift off easily, listing in my sleepy head all I received during the day and am grateful for, and thanking God for the opportunity to do it again tomorrow—because that alarm will soon be ringing.

22. Stress and You

How many aspects of your own life did you recognize in mine? The details may differ, but most of us juggle family, career, and social life and spend a fair amount of time just trying to keep our heads above water. Life is a daily slam that tests us to our very limits. How did this happen? Was it meant to be this way? Has it always been like this?

Interesting questions. No doubt people have felt stress for as long as there have been people. But the equation changed in some fundamental way fairly recently. A hundred years ago, life's stressors came rolling in like slow breakers on the ocean. You could often see them cresting on the horizon. If you worked on a farm, a drought would definitely be stressful, but it wouldn't sneak up on you like a job cut or a car accident. There was no twenty-four-hour TV barrage to worry you with how you should look or whether civil war halfway around the globe will affect you. Life has sped up quite a bit. Today, we worry about slow breakers rolling in much less than we do about riptides ready to suck us under at any moment.

Blame the speed of cars and planes for this change, and the instant communication made possible by TVs, phones, and E-mail. But don't forget the other change that swept the rug out from under women and left us on unfamiliar ground. After World War II, women slowly but surely broke out of house arrest and began having careers of their own. It's been an uphill battle—certain areas of business are still a man's world, and, on average, women earn only 76 percent of what their male colleagues make—but the women's movement has made great strides. Today women expect—and are expected—to have careers. Very good things came from this change, but hiding in that gift package were some unexpected challenges.

To pick up the slack for the household chore time lost when women entered the job market, men cut back on their hours, spent more time washing dishes and doing laundry, and began giving birth to half the babies.

No, wait, that's not what happened! Men's work hours have actually gone up, leaving them even less time to take care of kids or do household chores. As for making babies, call me if you've heard any miracle stories. Yes, in some ways it seems like somebody pulled a fast one on us. "Sure, you can have a career. Go for it! Just make sure you get dinner on the table and pick up the living room." "Sick kid? Guess you'll have to stay home today." "Yes, you can have a maternity leave, but while you're away, I'm going to give that promotion to Bob."

Don't get me wrong. I don't blame men for this situation. They are working harder than ever, too. In 1998, one in ten workers put in more than forty hours per week; now that number is one in four. And most husbands really do try to contribute to child rearing and even cooking more than their fathers did, but the fact is that the majority of housework still falls to women. And if things aren't working out at home, it usually isn't the man who is expected to ease off on his career. Somehow the system changed. Where one income was once just barely enough to have a house, two cars, a decent education for the kids, and all the necessities of life, now it takes two incomes to squeeze by.

This situation means that women today are stretched thinner than a piece of saltwater taffy. We're left feeling like we're getting closer and closer to that breaking point. And we're right—the stresses we feel really can break us in a million ways. Stress is not an irritation; it is a killer. Stress is closely linked with high blood pressure, heart disease, diabetes, stroke, ulcers, intestinal disorders, immune system collapse, autoimmune diseases, depression, migraines, asthma, sexual dysfunction, infertility, memory loss, and aging.

That's the bad news. The good news is that, even in the whirlwind of modern life, many strategies exist both to avoid stress and to reduce its impact when it does come. The challenge is greater than ever before, but with a little work, we can still create lives where stress becomes constructive, not destructive.

Yet even as we see the need to do something to relieve stress, we don't have a clear picture of exactly what stress is. Why do we feel it? And how can it affect us so powerfully?

What Is Stress?

Stress is simply demand placed upon something. The walls of your house experience stress from the weight of your roof upon them. There is nothing wrong with this, because they are up to the task. This is a normal, reasonable stress for them. If, on the other hand, a flying elephant decided to land on your roof, your walls might be in trouble. They would experience unreasonable stress and break down.

We work the same way, but in living beings, stress is also what promotes growth. When muscles and bones experience the normal stress of having to lift objects or move the body around, they respond by growing bigger and stronger so they can handle more stress next time. That's why strength training works. If muscles never experience demand on them, they shrink away to nothing.

Mental stress follows the same patterns. Children mature intellectually and emotionally by having normal demands placed upon them—demands they can handle. From cleaning up their rooms and learning to read to solving algebra equations and coping with the awkwardness of first dates, they grow into strong adults by dealing with constant, normal stress.

Pressure a five-year-old to try algebra, however, and she will act like those walls under the weight of the elephant: She will crack. Too much stress, whether physical or emotional, causes the same results.

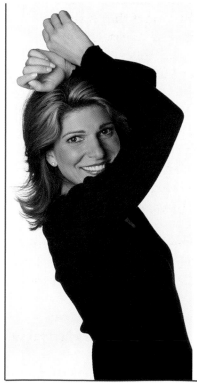

In fact, we don't really need to differentiate between physical and mental stress, because the body reacts to both with the same response. This is because the body first developed the stress response to deal with physical stress. Mental stress was a rarity back then. If we take a look at how the body reacts under stress, this makes perfect sense.

Cavemen didn't spend much time giving business presentations or interviewing for jobs, but they did have to run from predators, pursue game, compete with one another, and deal with food shortages or bad weather. Forty thousand years later, our bodies are still perfectly designed for such stressors. Think about your reactions to a stressful situation. Whether it's a boss yelling at you or a narrowly avoided traffic accident, your heart rate increases, you breathe more rapidly, and you feel hyperalert. This is the classic "fight or flight" response, and it doesn't work very well on a boss.

You can't karate-chop him, much as you might want to. Hightailing it out of the building doesn't work very well, either, if you want to hold on to your job.

If your problem is a saber-toothed tiger, however, these changes are just what you need. As soon as your body perceives some threat, it sends chemical messengers, called hormones, throughout your body. Like Paul Revere on his famous ride, the message these hormones deliver is, "The British are coming! Drop everything you're doing and deal with this immediately!" And your body does. It drops all long-term projects and concentrates its resources on surviving the next few minutes. This means diverting all available energy to the things you need to escape or fight—your limb muscles, your senses, and your brain. As we saw earlier, your energy comes from food, stored as sugar in your muscle or as fat on your body. When the stress hormones send out their alert, these fat stores get liquidated right away. They flood into your bloodstream, and your heart cranks up to several times its normal rate so it can pump them to your muscles as fast as possible. To convert this fat to energy, you need extra oxygen as well, so your lungs start working like crazy, too.

Dieters alert! Some of you may have read the above paragraph and thought, Aha! So stress causes me to liquidate my fat supply. To lose weight, I'm going to sneak into the zoo each night and let the polar bears chase me around! Yes, intense stress will cause you to lose weight, but you'll bounce right back when the stress disappears. And while chronic stress will definitely shave off the pounds, all that will do is help you fit into a skinnier coffin. Read on.

In addition to channeling extra energy to your muscles so you can run faster and swing harder, your body raises your senses to high alert. Your pupils dilate; your hearing perks up. This makes sense, because even better than running fast when that tiger is at your heels is hearing the tiger and climbing a tree while he's still crouching in the grass. A stick crunching in the night is still all it takes to send us into full stress response, eyes wide, heart slamming in our chest, thighs trembling with energy.

So far, so good. But already you start to see the problem. Using our big brains, we've gotten very good at anticipating trouble. Not only does the charging tiger set us off but the breaking stick that *might* be a tiger does, too. And why stop there? We are touring the jungle; our guide says, "This is tiger country." And *boom:* full response. A strange noise in the house at night and we are flicking on lights, heart racing as we try to wake that snoring husband to deal with the imaginary intruders.

The point to keep in mind is that a threat doesn't have to be real—or physical—to set us off. Anything we perceive as a threat or competition will do. A three-mile traffic jam works quite nicely, thank you. Or a coworker who undermines us. Or a big bill. Or the simple thought of public humiliation for any reason. The thought of a threat to our children ("It's two o'clock in the morning and the car's not home yet!") is one of the best ways to get a powerful stress response going, because not so long ago we mothers had to gear up to fight off whatever wanted to eat our little ones.

One problem with our stress response is that there are simply too many things to set it off in the modern world. In the days of cavemen, maybe people had to flee a predator once a year. Threats of starvation happened now and then. But the rest of the days, they ambled along, gathering nuts and berries, building fires, weaving clothing. Today, of course, threats—real and imaginary—come flying at us every hour of every day.

Another problem stems from the physical results of that stress. Our bodies are primed for action—muscles quivering, heart forcing huge amounts of blood through our system—but more often than not in the modern world, we *can't* react physically. If you're stuck in a traffic jam, the best you can do is turn up the radio and scream. If you're stuck in a meeting, the best you can do is kick the guy next to you.

I bet you see where I'm going with this. We get hit with stressors all the time, stressors that make our bodies shout, Run away! Fight! Get moving! So the very best way to ease this high-stress feeling is to do exactly what our bodies want: get moving. It's a whole lot healthier for your car to be driven at sixty-five miles per hour down the highway than for you to be revving its engine while stuck in neutral in the driveway.

Exercise burns away stress like nothing else. A couple of miles of walking and I've left that tiger way back in Pleistocene times. My body is relieved and can go back to its normal state. It even feels pain less. Exercise—as well as stress—floods the body with hormones called endorphins, which block the ability to sense pain. Very useful if a tiger is taking a swat at my backside; this also explains why I feel that nice "runner's high" after a good walk.

When I don't exercise, however, I'm stuck with those stress hormones surging through my body with no outlet. Not just the hormones, either: The fat that was released from my fat stores is circulating like mad, waiting to be converted into muscle energy, but if I don't need the muscle energy, the fat gets trapped in my bloodstream, where it is more likely to stick to artery walls. The extra pressure from my heart pounding all that blood through my arteries also tends to wear out the arteries, allowing blockages to form. This is why stress has such a huge effect on all the cardiovascular conditions and diseases helped by exercise—heart disease, high blood pressure, high cholesterol, diabetes, and stroke.

And that's just the beginning. Not a single body system is unaffected by stress. Remember how I said that stress hormones tell the body to forget any long-term projects and concentrate on surviving the immediate future? This means that as muscle power, heart rate, and perception get cranked up, everything else gets shut down. Digestion, for starters. Those blueberries in your stomach might make excellent fuel in a few hours, but if that tiger on your tail catches you, it hardly matters whether they get digested right now or not. Your immune system changes, too, sending all available forces to protect against yucky tiger germs that might soon be entering your system. Searching the rest of your body for garden-variety viruses and cancer cells is a luxury your immune system doesn't think it has under stress. (If stress gets chronic, your immune system may shut down entirely. Your body decides things are so dire that it can't expend energy on anything except running.)

Reproduction shuts down, too. Thinking about making a future generation only makes sense if you have a future. Under stress, both men and women experience less interest in sex. Women are less likely to get pregnant—their bodies show no interest until the stressors have passed. If getting pregnant is one of your goals, make sure your partner gives you as relaxed and stress-free an environment as possible.

Growth is another long-term project that can go by the wayside until stress is resolved. For adults, this means muscles wither, bones weaken, and tissues go unrepaired. We've all seen the effect of long-term stress on friends or family members. We watch their bodies get frail, hair turn gray, and skin lose its vigor. Stress, in fact, *is* aging in many ways. For kids, the effect is much worse, because they are still in the process of growing healthy bodies. Stress can curtail that growth.

By now, you get the picture of how terrible the effects of too much stress are on the body. But a few of you out there may still be seeing stress as a road to thinness, so I want to make the digestive facts very clear. When hit with immediate stress, digestion stops and appetite disappears. For the moment, your body couldn't care less about food. Any food that is in your stomach at the time just sits there.

But what happens when that stressor goes away? Your body dumped all those hard-earned fat and sugar supplies into your bloodstream so they could be used by your muscles for energy. Now that the tiger has been left in the dust, your body thinks it has to load up for the next emergency! You get ravenous, slapping every cookie within reach into your mouth. That's why so many people find that stress causes them to overeat—not during the stressful event, but soon after. So forget about losing weight through stress—unless you are planning on chronic 24/7 stress, in which case *see above* regarding stroke, heart disease, aging, and so on.

Still not convinced? Then think about how your stomach feels about being shut down with a pile of half-digested food in it. If this happens a few times a month, no problem. If it happens every day, things start to go wrong. The lining that protects your stomach from the powerful acids it uses to digest doesn't get fully replaced, and ulcers form. The bowels don't much like the on-off-on treatment, either; the result can be colitis or irritable bowel syndrome.

Okay, have I now made it clear that too much stress really stinks, and that we should do everything in our power to avoid it if we want to live long and well? Good. But that was the easy part. The hard part is figuring out what to do about it, because stress in the modern world is impossible to avoid. You just can't do it unless you want to go live as a yogi on top of a mountain, and even then you'd have your issues (cold, sunburn, birds landing on you). For the rest of us, the challenge is to design our lives to reduce exposure to stress in the first place and then to learn ways to deal efficiently with the stress we do feel.

WAYS TO REDUCE YOUR STRESS EXPOSURE

Don't get overwhelmed by the following tips. As with all other parts of my program, take this in small steps. Pick two or three things to try. Once you have those working, you can keep adding more techniques until you feel your stress is under control.

- **Turn off the TV and cancel the newspaper.** Amazing how many of us feel the need to worry about flooding in India, bulk milk prices in Wisconsin, and all the other far-flung stories the media foists on us every day. Almost everything you see on the news or hear about on the radio is beyond your control, and 95 percent of it seems to be negative. This adds more stress to your life than you may realize. If you are feeling overwhelmed, try cutting off these constant sources of doom and gloom. You may sleep a whole lot better.
- **Don't rush.** Being late for work and getting stuck in traffic may just be *the* definition of stress. Nothing gets the blood pressure rising faster. Even if you don't get stuck in traffic, if you are one of those people who is always ten minutes late and thus spends half the day dashing around, dressing on the way out the door, and wondering where the heck the keys are, you can do your body a tremendous favor by planning ahead, getting up fifteen minutes earlier, and saving yourself the constant worry of wondering whether you'll get somewhere on time. Doing this step will enable you to incorporate the next stress-busting tip.
- **Drive slower.** Unless you are on a cross-country marathon, driving ten miles per hour faster is not going to make a noticeable dent in your travel time. It's just going to make you worry about getting a ticket. Take it easy, enjoy the view, and (brace yourself) let other people get in front of you once in awhile.
- **Get rid of your cell phone.** Being on call to the world all day, every day, is a great way to get an ulcer. There are now these brilliant inventions that allow you to funnel all your calls to your home, where they will be saved up for you to review at your leisure. They are called answering machines. Try one. (Or at least keep your cell phone off when not making a call.)
- **Delegate.** This is one of the hardest tasks for us to learn—but one of the most valuable. I know that as my WalkAerobics business grew, I had to learn to trust others more and more. Too often we get stuck thinking, I'm the only one who knows how to do this. Even if that's true, eventually you'll get stretched too thin and crash. And remember: There was a time when you didn't know how to do it, either. You learned, and so can others. The more you delegate, the more you'll discover the power of enabling others. Soon you will be surrounded by

competent allies who will do all those boring things you used to think you needed to do. (Warning! If you are one of those people who doesn't delegate because, deep down, you think there is power in hoarding all the knowledge yourself, I've got a wake-up call for you. Not only is worrying about protecting your power base a fast track to a nervous breakdown—at which point someone's going to take over your job anyway—but it doesn't impress the leaders in your organization, either. The more power you give away, the more you will be trusted, and the more your leadership qualities will surface.)

- **Learn to say no.** Much of our stress load comes from our own good intentions: "Yes, I can have that report on your desk by Monday." "Yes, we'll come to your barbecue on Sunday." "Yes, I'll join the school board." "Yes, the whole basketball team can come over after school." Of course you want to do as much as you can for other people—that's a great quality—but if you commit to things you can't deliver, or say yes to so many commitments that your stress level zooms out of control and you become a truly unpleasant person to be around, then you aren't doing anybody any favors. Learn to say no politely and watch your accomplishments soar—and your stress plunge.

- **Break up tasks into doable chunks.** We all know the scenario: You get assigned some towering project at work. You're excited, but as you get into it, you realize just how immense it is. Then the mind games start. How am I ever going to do this? you wonder. What if I fail? I'll get fired. I'll lose the house. This is another case of letting your head get too far into the future. All you can do is one thing at a time, so break up the task into pieces and knock them out one by one. Usually, you'll find that you can do it, but if the task really is too much for one person, let others know up front, before it is too late. And *delegate!*

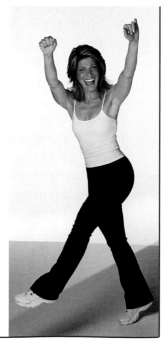

- **Avoid poisonous people.** Some people just stress you out. You know who they are. Either they are stressed themselves, and their agitation spills over to you, or they know how to push your buttons and do it for their own reasons. You can't let them do this. Ask them not to. If they persist, cross them off your list. You get only one life to live; don't let others mess it up.

- **Change jobs.** All of the stressors mentioned so far could be work-related. If you face a killer commute, if you have insane amounts of work piled on you and have no one to help you out, if your boss likes to see you sweat, or if you are just dealing with stressful material, you may want to consider a job change. That's a big step, so try other routes to alleviate the situation first. Talk problems over with your boss or the personnel office. See if you can adjust your job description to reduce your stress load. But if your company won't help you out, remind yourself that you come before they do.

- **Unclutter your environment.** By this, I *don't* mean doing dishes or picking up clothes—don't let chores get in the way of your walks! But a lot of us have "busy" environments, with TVs and cell phones beeping at us, music blaring, and houses crowded with furniture, toys, dusty exercise equipment, junk mail, and a million other things. We've forgotten the soothing feeling of being in simple, uncluttered, quiet spaces. Every piece of writing in a room, whether on posters, magazines, or computer screens, is something else competing for our attention. Turn the chatter down in your life by simplifying your home and office space, and you'll feel your stress level plummet.

- **Don't do your best.** I love this one, because it goes against what we hear all the time. Giving 110 percent is extremely stressful, because it means pushing yourself to the brink of collapse every time. Now and again, something comes up where it really does make sense to do your very best; the rest of the time, doing a good job is sufficient. Think back to those times in grade school when you scored ninety instead of one hundred. Now think how wildly different your life would be if you'd scored more one hundreds. That's right: not at all. Save the "do your best at any cost" mentality for the professional athletes and the overachievers who turn gray at thirty-five. This isn't an invitation to slack off; absolutely give everything you try a good effort, but don't get caught in the trap of always thinking, I could have done better. Enjoy your life a little.

- **Take breaks.** Too many hours of work without a break not only gets you wound up but makes you less productive, too. Take fifteen minutes every couple of hours to do . . . nothing. Walking makes a great break, of course, but so does closing your eyes and thinking about something as far away from work and home as possible. Do this and you'll find that you no longer slump during the second half of the day.

- **Stay away from caffeine.** I love my coffee, but it's a stressor, plain and simple. Caffeine and other stimulants crank up the stress response as surely as a saber-toothed tiger does. Your heart pounds, your breaths come fast, and your blood vessels constrict. If you drink only one or two cups a day, the stress is manageable, even helpful at times. But if you feel agitated during the day or aren't sleeping well at night, cut out the caffeine first thing.

- **Stay away from cigarettes.** They are a lousy stimulant anyway. I *hate* cigarettes. The only cigarette I ever smoked in my life was in Italy when I was eighteen. I'd gone over on a school trip and everyone there was smoking like a chimney. My girlfriends all picked up the habit, of course, and eventually they goaded me into trying one. *Nasty!* Never again. If you smoke, you are killing yourself for no good reason. Stop.

WAYS TO ALLEVIATE STRESS

So, you hired an assistant at work, began telecommuting two days a week, quit smoking, canceled your paper subscription, and you're *still* overstressed. Welcome to the club. Fortunately, the human race has spent the past several thousand years inventing some terrific ways to relax when the world is too much with us. Here are my favorites:

- **Exercise.** You know why. You know how. (Two tapes specifically focused on stress-reduction are my one-mile *Walk Away Your Stress* and *Evening Mile Plus Legs*.)
- **Unconditional love.** You love your kids deeply, even if they screw up, right? Now take that feeling and extend it to your spouse or parents. They aren't perfect, any more than you are, and if they do things that bug you, that says more about the stresses they are dealing with than it does about you. Give them the same kind of forgiving love you would a small child, even if you feel they don't deserve it. *Especially* if you feel they don't deserve it. Building up resentment only makes your life worse and adds to your stress level. Forgive, help them however you can, and feel the stress roll off your back. Then notice the way this changes your relationships with them. Once you've got this down, try extending the feeling to other family members and friends. Then push it out to acquaintances and, eventually, the whole world. It's good for the world, and it's even better for you.
- **The grandma game.** This is a simplified version of the unconditional love idea. Whenever somebody does something that gets your stress response going—cuts you off in traffic, can't find her purse in the supermarket checkout line—pretend that person is your grandmother (or grandson, or whatever it takes). Notice how this changes your response. That weary sympathy you'd have for an elderly relative is an excellent quality to cultivate. After all, the person probably *is* somebody's grandmother or grandson. Give them the benefit of the doubt.
- **Get distance.** When we feel threatened—somebody criticizes us at work, a family member shouts at us—our immediate instinct is to lash back. But instead of being defensive, try to distance yourself from your reaction immediately. Instead of thinking, How can I save face? think, What can we do to resolve the situation? You can even say this out loud. That immediately changes an adversarial situation into a partnership, with you and the other person working together to move forward.
- **Get religion.** More unconditional love. Studies show people with religious faith

are happier, experience less stress, and live longer than people who don't. If you haven't discovered what an incredible source of comfort God can be, you might want to check Him out.

- **Get out.** Social outlets reduce stress levels remarkably. Make sure you schedule regular evenings out with the girls to blow off steam, or join a club that appeals to you.
- **Get hitched.** People who are married or in long-term partnerships have lower stress levels than those who are single. They live longer, too. It just helps to have a shoulder to cry on now and then.
- **Get help.** If you feel like your stress level is becoming overwhelming, don't hesitate to find a therapist. Talking it all out with someone who knows the territory really can make a huge difference. If visiting a psychotherapist makes you uncomfortable, try talking with your minister or a really good friend.
- **Get in the mood.** What better way to roll your exercise and socializing into one? A tried-and-true stress reducer.
- **Get a massage.** Nothing makes you feel better than a massage. The relaxation, the relief from sore muscles, the gentle human touch are all wonderful. It's impossible to stay stressed during a massage. If I were president, I would make everyone get a daily massage—as long as they exercised!
- **Breathe easy.** It seems too simple to work, but just taking a deep breath triggers a cascade of stress reduction in your body. Because short breaths go along with the "fight or flight" response, a long, slow breath signals to the body that the danger has passed. It really works, and you can do it anywhere!
- **Take a bath.** Warm water and the lack of outside stimulus cause your muscles to relax, your breathing to slow, and your heart rate to drop. But you already know this.
- **Stretch.** Stress builds up in our muscles, especially in our shoulders, neck, and jaw. Give yourself some reminders at your desk to take a few minutes every hour to stretch. Stand up, and stretch those legs and arms. Then roll your head around until you feel the pressure easing along your neck. Then consciously unclench your jaw. Then notice how much better you work.
- **Light some candles.** Something about the age-old flickering of candlelight whisks us back to a time when the world moved more slowly, and so could we. Keep lots of candles on hand; they can be as essential to your health as good sneakers.
- **Listen to music.** Not just any music. Different types of music trigger different waves in the brain. Classical music with a beat similar to the resting human heart triggers alpha waves—slow brain patterns that occur during moments of deep relaxation, heightened awareness, and creativity. It also eliminates the faster beta waves generated during stress and anger. Slower music can induce the theta waves common during sleep. Every music store now has a section devoted

to healing music. Try some out. It's one of the best ways to unwind at the end of a tough day.

- **Try aromatherapy.** Aromatherapy is the science of how scents affect the brain. Certain scents relax you. Lavender and jasmine are two of the best. You can pick from many different essential oils and can buy an infuser for putting the scents into the air. Combine this stress-reduction technique with baths, candles, or massage for an evening of stress-banishing bliss.
- **Try yoga.** Don't be intimidated by it. It may seem exotic, but yoga is incredibly easy. Instructors are always offering introductory courses and are happy to have new recruits. The slow exercises of yoga were designed specifically to bring the body into a state of physical relaxation, mental alertness, and spiritual awareness. It really works! If you aren't ready to take a course yet, try my new video *You Can Do Yoga*. It's guaranteed to get you started in no time.
- **Laugh.** Oh, I feel a cliché coming on, but laughter really is the best medicine. It chases away those stress hormones and replaces them with feelin'-good endorphins. And it's contagious. Spread some today. If a garden-variety stressful event occurs, try seeing the humorous side of it. (As I suggested elsewhere, try seeing yourself as the lead in your own sitcom.) People who can laugh at themselves rarely get wrapped up in stress.
- **Dance.** Dance is really just a great way for a group of people to get exercise at once. You get all the health benefits of exercise, along with the extra stress reduction that comes from socializing. You usually end up laughing, too!
- **Keep a diary.** Having a place to spill your frustrations can be a wonderful release. Not only do you get it all out but then you have a way of going over it all in a more objective manner once you've cooled down. You can use your fitness journal for this purpose, or if you prefer a completely blank book, you'll find many different styles in all good bookstores, card shops, and art-supply stores.
- **Take a vacation.** Anything—and anybody—starts to grate after awhile. Make sure you get occasional breaks—from your job, your house, and, yes, even from your family. Escape for a weekend with a favorite girlfriend. You'll enjoy your regular life a lot more when you get back—and the people in your life will thank you for it.

23. The Motivation Station

In one sense, this chapter is a tool to support the walking program in this book. In another, it stands on its own and can be used in ways that have nothing to do with walking. The kind of motivation I recommend requires you to do no more and no less than change the entire way you view yourself and the world. Whether this is the hardest or easiest thing you've ever done depends on how tenaciously you hold on to negative beliefs.

There are different kinds of motivation in the world. There is drill sergeant motivation. If you rely on someone screaming in your face, commanding you to get up and walk, it will work just fine—until the day you leave the army. This and all the other fear motivators—fear of punishment, of disease if you don't exercise, of ridicule—tend to backfire over time. As soon as the threat is removed, you tend to slip—especially since you have built up resentment toward the fear motivator and want to rebel at some level.

Somewhat more effective than fear motivators are reward motivators: the carrot instead of the stick. These have their place; at the very least, you learn to associate the activity with the pleasant rewards. The rewards don't have to be material, either. Children are motivated to do all sorts of good things—picking up their rooms, saying please and thank you, even learning new skills—by the praise they receive from adults. As I said, this can be effective, and it's a necessary part of life. The trouble comes if we learn this lesson too well and grow up still looking to some external source for our motivation.

Not that motivation from within is perfect, either. You can be your own drill sergeant, or you can come up with all sorts of mental self-torture to force yourself into action. One common yet misguided piece of advice we receive is to use willpower to achieve our goals. Captains of industry write their memoirs and self-help books, explaining how they rose to the top and routed the competition through sheer force of will, and how you can do the same. Well, willpower is certainly an important quality, and there do seem to be a few people out there like Michael Jordan who can accomplish anything they want through willpower alone, but for the rest of us mere mortals, pure willpower eventually breaks down. If I don't really want to exercise but I set myself a goal of exercising every day because "That is what I am going to do," there always comes a day when I can't force myself out of bed, when the sheer effort involved is more than I can overcome.

What I need instead is a situation where achieving my goal—whether it's exercise, quitting smoking, or anything else—does not require superhuman effort or a self-imposed pep talk. What I need is a situation where success is easy. I'm going to teach you how to set up just such a situation, where the initial desire comes from within but your whole environment helps motivate you by reinforcing good behavior and limiting your access to bad choices.

We tend to resist this idea because we have it ingrained in us that the desire to change must come from within and that external motivators are somehow inauthentic. True, the desire to change starts inside. If you don't have that, then no amount of external influence will make a difference. But so many of us have the desire, yet we haven't been able to achieve success. Every failed crash diet attests to this. That's because too often we are fighting an uphill battle in a world set against us succeeding, because we have underestimated the power of our environment to influence our behavior. But, as more behavioral psychologists are learning, change the environment and you really can transform the person.

New York City is a terrific example. In the 1970s and 1980s, New York was riddled with crime. Everything, from robbery and drug use to murder, was spiraling out of control. More prisons and tougher sentences (motivation by punishment) had no impact. In the 1990s, with a limited budget for law enforcement, Mayor Rudolph Giuliani's administration tried a different approach. They focused hard on the minor but conspicuous crimes, like jaywalking, shoplifting, and vandalism. They scrubbed graffiti from subway cars and fixed broken windows. They gave the city a

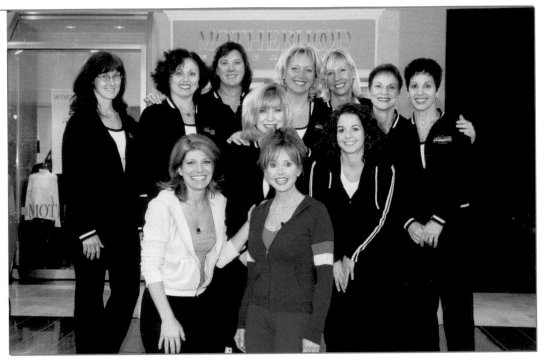
Nothing gets me motivated like my amazing walking team!

feeling of order, cleanliness, and security. Many people ridiculed them, but the plan succeeded beyond anyone's dreams. Not only did the number of petty crimes plunge but even violent crimes took a nosedive. New York City's murder rate was cut by *two-thirds* in only five years.

What had happened? Had half the criminals in New York suddenly moved out because there was no more graffiti on the walls? Of course not. The same people who would have committed violent crimes in the past were now being law-abiding citizens, and the only thing that had changed was the city's sense of orderliness. In some powerful way, the city's environment now made crime less thinkable. The people who would have been committing crimes in the past were either not getting the idea any more or were not acting on the idea if they did get it. Through subtle cues, their environment reinforced good behavior.

How does this apply to us? Well, if our surroundings encourage it, most of us have the potential to be "criminal" to ourselves—not exercising, eating poorly, and doing all the other things that hurt us down the road. Rather than getting down on ourselves for what we think of as our weaknesses, we can solve many of these problems simply by setting up our environment for success.

This is a pretty revolutionary idea. Tell someone that being fit or out of shape has more to do with her home, neighborhood, friends, and job than with her personality and you are likely to get a raised eyebrow. It sounds like you're looking for excuses, for someone to blame. But there isn't anyone to blame, because, as adults, we have every opportunity to change our environment. The only person to blame is ourselves if we don't take the simple steps needed to ensure our own success.

If this seems like a strange idea to you, think about spas. Spas, substance-abuse centers, and weight-loss "farms" are all built on the idea that most of us can become healthy if surrounded by a healthy environment. Put someone in a beautiful setting with a multitude of exercise options, access to nothing but health food, and—most important of all—other people doing the same thing, and that person will get fit. Success is easy. Unfortunately, this environment is temporary. When you get released back into the real world, the bad behaviors usually return.

My idea of permanent, powerful motivation is to turn your whole life into a "spa environment," but to do it on a tiny budget—moneywise and timewise. Bill Gates can build a real spa in his house and take whatever time off he needs; you need to figure out how to create that same kind of spa environment, where healthy options are always at hand and temptation is nonexistent, and then fit it into your existing family and work life.

In a way, that's what *Walk Away the Pounds* is all about. You may have noticed how these ideas underlie all the concepts I've introduced in this book. Most people fail to exercise not because they are lazy at heart but because they don't have the time to drive to a fitness club, are intimidated by the exercises done there, or work too many hours and can't figure out how to squeeze the exercise in. In-home walking goes a long way to creating a fail-safe environment because it eliminates the obstacles of time, distance, and difficulty. I hope my Walk Diet goes even further than that. The goal is to make walking an integral part of your life. That way it is not just something you do; it is part of who you are. At this level, motivation becomes effortless, like breathing. We're strongly motivated to breathe, too, but few of us have to remind ourselves to do it.

That's why it is so important to get past that twenty-one-day stage, where new habits are formed. Once walking becomes a habit, you no longer have to force yourself to do it. Ditto for eating healthy, thinking positive thoughts, or any other behavior. Here, then, is my no-fail ten-step motivation program. Use it to achieve amazing and effortless results in anything you attempt.

STEP ONE: MAKE IT DOABLE

Whatever your goal, if you make it something way beyond your capabilities, you aren't doing yourself any favors. You won't achieve it, you'll get discouraged, and you'll give up. If we stick a three-year-old on a bike and tell him to ride, he's going to crash and then won't be very keen on riding for a long time. Make your immediate goal something you know you can do. Despite what generations of high school coaches have taught us, don't "leave it all on the playing field." Don't push yourself to the brink of exhaustion. Just do a good job, and then do a slightly better job when you're ready. Eventually, you will achieve goals that at first seemed beyond you. Remember that proverb about the man who lifted his calf every day, and as the calf grew up, the man was able to keep on lifting it!

STEP TWO: GET IN YOUR FACE

The very best way to do something regularly is to have constant reminders to do it. It should be so present that you almost can't avoid it. If the Walk Diet is your goal, then you want walking shoes at home *and* at work (or shoes that double as work/walking shoes—they do exist), tapes at home and a DVD for your office computer, and a chart on your fridge, reminding you each morning of your daily goal. Don't bury the tapes in the bottom of your TV cabinet, either. Put them right on top between two bookends. One great tool for staying focused on your goals is an exercise journal. Using it will also keep those goals in sight (see Step Four).

STEP THREE: SEEK OUT POSITIVE PEOPLE

As a parent, I know that the crowd my children hang out with has a huge influence on their behavior. My kid may have excellent internal values, but if his entire crowd is shoplifting and telling him he's a loser if he doesn't do it, he is going to need incredible willpower to resist the pressure. Same goes for adults and exercise or poor eating. If your friends believe that exercise is a waste and are interested only in watching TV or going out for dessert, you are going to be forcing yourself to exercise alone. Staying away from bad food means missing out on your social life. That's a tough spot to be in. Cultivate new friends, people who like to exercise, and suddenly exercise feels much easier. You don't have to make yourself do it; you *want* to do it. You don't want to miss out on the fun. And if you know friends are stopping by at eight o'clock in the morning to do a walking tape with you, you'll be much less likely to cancel than if you are on your own. Get to this point and you're golden. On my Web site, you can find other walkers in your area and join a group. You *know* they'll be dedicated.

In addition to being actual exercise partners, friends can either support you or undercut you in more subtle ways. Friends and family members who notice the differences in you each week and comment on how much closer to your goal you are can help tremendously. People who put down your walking program and suggest that you skip it are poisoning your motivation. Explain to them that you need their support. If they don't change, and they are friends or coworkers, they can be avoided. You can't avoid your family, but you can make it very clear to them how important this is to you.

Don't forget the value of "virtual" support, too. Books, tapes, and Web sites can all contribute to weaving a community of helpers around you and setting up an environment that constantly reminds you to stay on task.

STEP FOUR: COMMIT IT TO WRITING

The mind is a trickster. You can have the best intentions in the world, can even recite them to yourself each morning, but then a funny thing happens as time passes. You don't want to walk one morning, cite poor sleep as an excuse, and then at the end of that week, when you've only walked four times instead of five, you tell yourself that's still pretty good. Soon three times a week is still pretty good, and your intentions are to get in three good walks. You don't even remember your goal of five walks a week. You aren't lying to yourself; the mind just has a way of fudging as it needs to. How many New Year's resolutions have we made, fully intending to keep them, and then a few weeks later they disappear from our thoughts entirely? That's why it's vital to write down your goals. Putting them down on paper makes them real and unalterable; you know clearly whether you've met them or not. Of course, committing them to paper and then burying the paper in some drawer doesn't help, either. Use a journal to develop your goals and check it every day. That way, you'll fulfill Step Two: keeping your goals in your face.

STEP FIVE: A LIFE-AFFIRMING BELIEF SYSTEM

It astonishes me how many people choose to believe that life is meaningless, that there is nothing beyond the basic reality we see. Not only is there no evidence to support this but the impoverished spirit it leaves you with is a terrible burden to have to carry around. By searching inside yourself until you touch that sacred spark that *knows* you are connected to everything else in this universe, you gain access to the greatest motivator you will ever find: the knowledge that you belong in this world, as surely as your finger belongs to you, and that the love that suffuses the world is pushing you to be active, healthy, and happy. If you believe there is something sacred about the stars, about the sky, about Niagara Falls, then you must accept that there is something sacred about you, too. Don't try to reason this out. That's not your job. Just feel it and live it. Be it. *That's* your job.

STEP SIX: AVOID TEMPTATION

Oscar Wilde said it best: "I can resist everything except temptation." Who can? But the solution is simple: Make your house your sanctuary. Whatever your bad habit, get everything related to it as far from your life as possible. If you do, you'll be cured. A smoker who is stranded on a desert island without that daily pack is no longer a smoker. Alcoholics who want to give up drinking don't apply for jobs in liquor stores. If your goal is to be fit and eat less junk, the best favor you can do yourself is to clear your house of junk food. First thing tomorrow, throw out all sweets of any kind. I don't just mean your kitchen cupboards, either. Hit your bedroom and the bowl of candy in the living room. Don't forget the glove compartment in your car and your office drawers. The goal is to remove temptation from all facets of your life. If you drive past a bakery with extraordinary cinnamon rolls on your way to work, change your route. Tell your friends not to bring sweets or snacks into the house. If it isn't there, you can't eat it.

Don't trick yourself into focusing solely on desserts. Muffins are just cake in disguise. Sodas, sugary breakfast cereals, and chips are all just as bad. Remove all these temptations from your life. Like bad boyfriends, you'll miss them at first, but after a few weeks you'll wonder what you ever saw in them in the first place.

I know, I know. But Leslie, you're thinking, I live in America. I *can't* remove fast-food restaurants from my roads. I have to stop for gas at convenience stores that are packed with Milky Ways. I can't control the whole world. True. Environment makes a huge difference in your actions, but ultimately it is still up to you. Short of chaining yourself to your bed, you can't create an environment where you are *unable* to give in to temptation. But bottled water, ready-to-go salads, and bags of pretzels are just as accessible as junk food. As I discussed earlier in this chapter, studies like the one of New York City's crime problem show that simple changes in external cues do make the difference for most people. And I'm willing to bet you're one of those people.

Having said that, I'll offer you another way out. If you feel that it is just impossible to remove or resist the temptations in your world, consider changing worlds. Drastic, I know, but the power of place is stronger than you think. If your goal is never again to touch a bratwurst and you live in Milwaukee, you're in trouble. If you move to Japan, success is guaranteed. If you feel that you won't achieve fitness unless you never again are confronted with a Whopper, move to the mountains of Wyoming—somewhere where the nearest fast-food chain is two hundred miles away. Geography can play a huge role in exercise behavior, too. If you hate cold weather and live in the Northeast, there are going to be a lot of months when you stay cooped up inside. (Thank goodness for indoor walking!) Move to Arizona and you may find yourself much more active. If swimming is your favorite exercise but you live in Kansas, you may discover a whole new person if you move to the Florida coast. If your favorite method of walking is from shop to shop, find a city with a great pedestrian marketplace where you can do your grocery and gift shopping on your feet. More and more cities have them.

STEP SEVEN: AVOID BRAINWASHING

This step is an extension of the temptation step. There is direct temptation—the box of doughnuts beckoning to you from the top of the fridge—and then there is the constant whispering in your ear from TV, billboards, and magazines, telling you that you need to drink what's cool, wear what's cool, and look a certain way. TV commercials pound brand names of sodas and chips into our heads, so that when we enter a supermarket, we shuffle toward the chip display like zombies, arms outstretched. Equally destructive is the media emphasis on being glitzy, whip-thin, and twenty-five years old for life. If you are really serious about developing healthy attitudes toward fitness, about detoxifying your environment, then you need to go beyond the immediate threats and remove the poisonous cues that surround you, too.

STEP EIGHT: RECOGNIZE NEGATIVE THINKING PATTERNS

I could devote an entire chapter to the pain we all inflict on ourselves through destructive thinking patterns. There are a million varieties, about which I'm sure you know plenty, but they all come down to the same issue: not existing in the here and now. If you can truly focus on the present moment, your choices become incredibly easy. If exercise is the issue, the question becomes: Will I be better off if I walk today? The answer is yes. The only way this gets complicated is when your mind starts bringing the past and future into it. Then the dangerous mind games start. See how many of these you recognize:

"What's the point in walking today? I'll only lose a quarter of a pound or so."

"I skipped yesterday, so even if I walk today, I won't be caught up to where I should be. It's hopeless; I blew it."

"If I walk twice tomorrow, I can skip today."

"I've tried ten diets and none of them has worked. What makes me think this will be any different?"

"When I've lost a hundred pounds, I'll look good."

"My parents were fat and I was meant to be, too. It doesn't matter what I try."

"I could walk from here to Timbuktu and I still wouldn't look like *her*."

"If I had started this a year ago, I'd really be showing progress now."

These thoughts, and many like them, lure you into the realm of daydreaming. They trick you into ignoring the one reality: that anything you do happens one step at a time, and you start from today.

That much is obvious. Less obvious is how fast negative thoughts can crackle through your brain. Once these patterns get established—and in many of us, they were established in early childhood—without even being conscious of it, we go from "I wish I was better at this" to "I'm not as good as other people," to "I may as well accept my sorry fate," to "I give up." We're not even aware of it. All we know is that at the first sign of struggle, our whole goal seemed hopeless.

If you suspect that negative thinking patterns hold you back in life, do some reverse detective work to find out. When you're hit with that feeling of hopelessness, self-criticism, or depression, ask yourself where that feeling came from. Track your thoughts backward over the past few minutes. See if you can remember what led to what. With practice, you may uncover some dysfunctional reasoning hiding out in your very own brain and hijacking it. (If you can't ferret out your thought patterns on your own, therapists can help tremendously.)

Your other alternative is not to worry about the negative thoughts, but to ignore them and keep yourself strongly focused on the here and now. All you have is today. What can you do to get the most out of it?

STEP NINE: NO SLIPS FOR FOUR WEEKS

As you now know, twenty-one days is the key to establishing a new habit. After that, your brain and body expect to do the new activity; you just have to follow through. Once the new habit is established, you can slip now and then and it won't affect your overall success or motivation. You'll get right back to it the next day. But earlier slips interfere with the formation of the new pattern. For the first four weeks, try extra hard to stick to your goals. If necessary, remind yourself that you *will* be allowed to deviate eventually. That should keep you from getting discouraged. Sticking to something with no slips for four weeks is doable; doing it *for life* with no slips isn't.

STEP TEN: REWARDS

Rewards can be two-edged swords. As I said earlier, becoming too attached to rewards can keep us from looking for satisfaction within ourselves or from enjoying an activity for itself. It can get us focused on the future, not the present. On the other hand, rewards can be powerful motivators. If used judiciously, they can work well as a stepping-stone to deeper motivators. So, if you find that the previous nine motivators haven't quite done the trick, see if rewards can push you over the top.

The trick with rewards is to keep them in proportion to the goal. If the goal is to walk two miles for the first time, the reward is not a new car. Small rewards on a daily basis help give you a good feeling about your activity without making the activity seem beside the point. Fresh flowers, new books, or a luxurious bath make good daily rewards. A different hairdo or new clothes could reward sticking to your goals for a week. When you reach big milestones, by all means reward yourself appropriately. Just make sure the rewards aren't detrimental to your goals. No candy if the goal is weight loss! No champagne if the goal is not drinking!

Try to keep the rewards and the activity closely linked. Pick a restaurant a couple of miles away from you and walk to it for dinner. Rent the new movie you've been dying to see and stick it under this book. Until you've lifted the book and done your walking routine, no touching the movie. Some people—people who really don't trust themselves—take this idea to extremes. If you think nothing else will do, park your car a mile away at a friend's house or a big parking lot. You can't go anywhere until you get to your car. I *guarantee* you'll get your walking in.

I like to use rewards in the Walk Diet subtly. They aren't the reason we exercise;

they just help to keep the whole process fun and cuddly. I think of them as a stopgap measure. They're a great way to get started, but after four weeks, I hope you'll be able to achieve your goals because you know they are good for you and you like to do them. At that point, daily rewards should drop away. Definitely treat yourself now and then, and always celebrate big milestones in style, but otherwise strike a balance between being good to yourself and expecting a lot from yourself.

Last Word: Be Absolutely Honest

Here you have the world's easiest motivation system, to go along with the world's easiest fitness system. Use it to get fit, use it to boost your career to the next level, or use it to reinvigorate your relationship. However you use it, I want you to know that you *can* fail with this system—but only if you really want to fail. You can write down your goals, pile walking tapes in your living room, hang around supportive friends, clear the junk food out of your house, and still cheat yourself by skipping your walk to drive to the nearest convenience store for three pints of chocolate fudge chunk ice cream. If you won't be honest with yourself, there's nothing I or anyone else can do to help you.

Know, however, that it's actually more work to cheat this system than to follow it. That's the whole point: Success is easier than failure. Still, if deep down you want to fail, if you are just fooling yourself about your desire to change, you can find a way. Some people will work amazingly hard at sabotaging themselves. That's why this last step, which could just as easily be Step One, is to be completely honest with yourself—and with everyone else. One thing I've learned in life is that even if it seems to make things harder immediately, honesty always makes your life easier in the long run. Before you go to the trouble of rearranging the externals in your life to reinforce your goals, make sure that's what you really want. If it is, everything else is doable.

24. Let Me Hear from You!

I've spent a bit of time in this book talking about the drawbacks of the Internet—the way it speeds up communication and adds to our stress levels. So let me take a moment to talk about one of the great qualities of the Internet: It allows you to reach out to others and create a community on-line. I've been working hard to create such a community, and you can join it at:

www.lesliesansone.com

I love logging on to the Web site and following the ongoing conversations there, seeing the way we support one another and draw strength from our common goals. I hope you will use the site to help you achieve your own walking goals. Here are a few ideas:

1. Find role models. When you begin the program, you can read about many more Walking Wonders like the ones you've read about in this book. You are bound to find some whose stories resonate strongly with you, and who can serve as inspiration for your own success.

2. Join my Walk Club. In this members-only area, you can:

• Participate in brand-new Walk Diets. I lead several a year.

• Get advice from personal trainers, motivation experts, dieticians—and me, of course!

• Find healthy, simple, and scrumptious recipes to keep you fit and energized.

• Join the conversation in live forums and chat rooms where others like you are sharing their stories, challenges, and success secrets.

3. Sign up for my free E-newsletter to keep up to date on all the developments in the world of in-home walking.

4. Keep the fun in walking—and keep progressing—by getting new products to liven up your workouts. In addition to all my videos and DVDs, you can get cassettes and CDs, hand weights, resistance bands, pedometers and heart-rate monitors, books and journals, dietary supplements, walk pants and sweats, and anything else you might need.

5. Get a fitness profile. Answer some simple questions about your body type, size, weight, age, and goals, and I'll give you a customized recommendation for the workouts best suited to your needs.

6. Send in your story. I love to hear the success stories of people who have used my program to turn their lives around. When you become one of those people, I want to know!

7. Learn about taking classes at Studio Fitness. If you really want to feel like a part of the family, you can take a trip to visit my amazing team of Walk Leaders and me at Studio Fitness in New Castle, Pennsylvania. We'll get you inspired!

8. Tell me anything at all. I adore feedback! Really, it means so much to me. It's what keeps me energized and loving life.

You don't have to be a Web surfer to be a part of our family, either. At Studio Fitness, we have wonderful real live people happy to help you out. Give us a call.

Studio Fitness
2801 Wilmington Road
New Castle, PA 16105
888-440-9255

Acknowledgments

To name and thank everyone who has been on this journey with me would take a BOOK in itself, so here's the short version.

To everyone at Studio Fitness: It's so much more than physical fitness . . . we have been walking the "Walk of Life" together and how blessed I am to receive so much love and support.

Thanks to QVC for allowing me to be the first-ever guest on the network.

Thanks to Goodtimes video family, and to the producers of my videos and TV spots.

Thanks to Nina for that brave "let's do something about it" spirit, in work and in life. And millions of thanks for finding Rowan! Rowan, you are my angel from God for making this book happen!

Thanks to Rolf and his team at Warner Faith for showing interest from the beginning, and to Diana and the Warner Books team for being so great to work with.

To my family, friends, and above all my Creator, who brings all meaning to life, I am forever grateful.

Resources

VIDEOS AND CDs

Leslie Sansone In-Home Walking
2801 Wilmington Road
New Castle, PA 16105
888-440-9255
www.lesliesansone.com

My videos can match all your walking needs, from one-mile beginner walks to four-mile PowerWalks. There are tapes, CD-ROMs, and DVDs that incorporate strength training, aerobics or yoga moves, faster-paced walks, and stretching. One of my favorites is the Walk the Walk series, which combines walking with uplifting music to bring you a little closer to God as you move. I also have CDs to motivate you through any walk, indoors or out. If you are out shopping, you can look for my products in Target, Wal-Mart, Kmart, Costco, Sam's Club, BJ's Warehouse, and elsewhere.

EQUIPMENT

My section on gear in chapter 4 covers the basics on shoes, clothing, weights, and other strength-training helpers. You can get everything but the shoes from my In-Home Walking store, and you can get everything including shoes at any good discount store. For some of the specialty walking shoes, you'll need to visit a shoe store.

MAGAZINES

Health
www.health.com

If you're sick of poisoning yourself with bad food and bad habits, *Health* will teach you everything you need to know about good food, safe environments, exercise benefits, and other ways to live the good life.

Prevention
www.prevention.com

Health news, recipes, workouts, and more appear in every issue.

Weight Watchers Magazine
www.weightwatchers.com
　The ideal magazine to support your weight-loss commitment.

Woman's Day
www.womansday.com
　My favorite magazine for the modern woman, filled with great health tips, style coverage, recipes, fitness routines, career information, and ideas for alleviating stress.

Web Sites and Organizations

American Heart Association
www.americanheart.org
800-242-8721
　If you have any heart concerns, this is the place to take them. You'll learn the facts on heart health, discover programs that will help you stay healthy and active, and find information on local events.

Andrew Weil
www.drweil.com
　Dr. Weil is our leading expert on healing through healthy lifestyle. His emphasis on exercise, healthy diet, stress reduction, natural foods, and vitamins is a breath of fresh air in our overmedicated world. His Web site is the best source for information on natural health, and his "Vitamin Advisor" link offers customized multivitamins.

Cooper Aerobics Center
www.cooperaerobics.com
800-444-5192
　Dr. Kenneth Cooper is known as "the Father of Aerobics." He is also one of my personal heroes. More than any other person, Dr. Cooper is responsible for putting aerobic exercise on the map. His 1968 best-seller, *Aerobics*, got the exercise trend started, and he has followed that up with a string of best-sellers teaching us about the importance of keeping the body moving, including *The New Aerobics*, *Aerobics for Women*, *Fit Kids*, and *Faith-Based Fitness*. His Cooper Aerobics Center in Dallas, Texas, spearheads cutting-edge research on fitness and health, and his Wellness Center is one of the premier spas in the nation. His Web site is a great resource for everything from health information to ordering Cooper Complete, Dr. Cooper's specially formulated multivitamin.

Florine Mark

The WW Group, Inc.

www.florineonline.com

Florine Mark, founder of many of the Weight Watchers franchises in the Midwest and on the East Coast, is one of the most amazing motivational speakers you'll ever meet. I love partnering with this inspiring woman. Log on to her Web site for advice, motivation, and to be part of a great community.

Jenny Craig

www.jennycraig.com

800-597-5366

With an emphasis on healthy choices and emotional balance, Jenny Craig has been helping people gain control over their eating for many years. On the Web site, you can find recipes, support, success stories, local franchise information, and much more.

Weight Watchers

www.weightwatchers.com

The premier weight-loss organization in the country, Weight Watchers has helped millions of people lose weight over the past forty years by encouraging healthy eating, community support, and fitness. You can find the local franchise in your neighborhood through the national Web site or by looking in your phone book.

Body Mass Index Table

No matter how overweight you are, losing as little as five pounds can reduce your risk of disease. But true long-term health comes when you stay within a target area of healthy weights. To pinpoint these weights, the Body Mass Index (BMI) table was developed. It lists healthy weights for people of different heights. Healthy BMIs are between 18.5 and 25. Above 25, you increase your risk of diabetes, cardio-vascular disease, and certain cancers. Above 30, your chance of these diseases skyrockets.

To use the table, find your height in the left-hand column. Move across to your weight. The number at the top of the column is your BMI.

BMI	19	20	21	22	23	24	25	26	27	28	29	30	31	32	33	34	35
Height (inches)					**Body Weight (pounds)**												
58	91	96	100	105	110	115	119	124	129	134	138	143	148	153	158	162	167
59	94	99	104	109	114	119	124	128	133	138	143	148	153	158	163	168	173
60	97	102	107	112	118	123	128	133	138	143	148	153	158	163	168	174	179
61	100	106	111	116	122	127	132	137	143	148	153	158	164	169	174	180	185
62	104	109	115	120	126	131	136	142	147	153	158	164	169	175	180	186	191
63	107	113	118	124	130	135	141	146	152	158	163	169	175	180	186	191	197
64	110	116	122	128	134	140	145	151	157	163	169	174	180	186	192	197	204
65	114	120	126	132	138	144	150	156	162	168	174	180	186	192	198	204	210
66	118	124	130	136	142	148	155	161	167	173	179	186	192	198	204	210	216
67	121	127	134	140	146	153	159	166	172	178	185	191	198	204	211	217	223
68	125	131	138	144	151	158	164	171	177	184	190	197	203	210	216	223	230
69	128	135	142	149	155	162	169	176	182	189	196	203	209	216	223	230	236
70	132	139	146	153	160	167	174	181	188	195	202	209	216	222	229	236	243
71	136	143	150	157	165	172	179	186	193	200	208	215	222	229	236	243	250
72	140	147	154	162	169	177	184	191	199	206	213	221	228	235	242	250	258
73	144	151	159	166	174	182	189	197	204	212	219	227	235	242	250	257	265
74	148	155	163	171	179	186	194	202	210	218	225	233	241	249	256	264	272
75	152	160	168	176	184	192	200	208	216	224	232	240	248	256	264	272	279
76	156	164	172	180	189	197	205	213	221	230	238	246	254	263	271	279	287

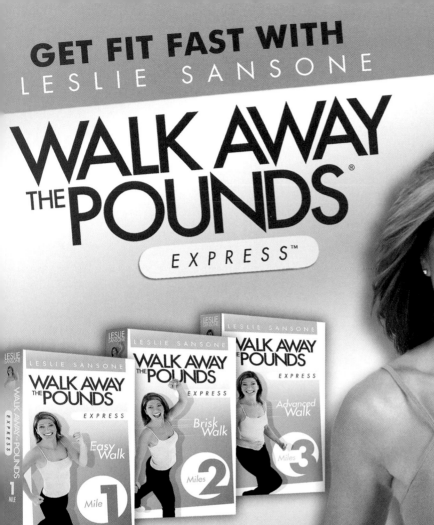